VI
Nursing Management of Adults With Urinary Problems

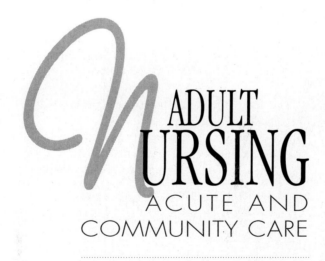

ADULT
NURSING
ACUTE AND
COMMUNITY CARE

SECOND EDITION

Burrell • Gerlach • Pless

Copyright © 1997 by Appleton & Lange
A Simon & Schuster Company
Copyright © 1992 by Appleton & Lange
A Publishing Division of Prentice Hall

97 98 99 00 01/ 10 9 8 7 6 5 4 3 2 1

Prentice Hall International (UK) Limited, *London*
Prentice Hall of Australia Pty. Limited, *Sydney*
Prentice Hall Canada, Inc., *Toronto*
Prentice Hall Hispanoamericana, S.A., *Mexico*
Prentice Hall of India Private Limited, *New Delhi*
Prentice Hall of Japan, Inc., *Tokyo*
Simon & Schuster Asia Pte. Ltd., *Singapore*
Editora Prentice Hall do Brasil Ltda., *Rio de Janeiro*
Prentice Hall, *Upper Saddle River, New Jersey*

Please send suggestions and comments about *Adult Nursing: Acute and Community Care,* ed. 2 to Lenette O. Burrell at School of Nursing/Athens, Medical College of Georgia, 1905 Barnett Shoals Road, Athens, GA 30605.

Library of Congress Cataloging-in-Publication Data

Adult Nursing : acute and community care / [edited by] Lenette Owens
  Burrell, Mary Jo M. Gerlach, Betsy S. Pless. — 2nd ed.
      p. cm.
  Rev. ed. of: Adult nursing in hospital and community settings.
  c1992.
  Includes bibliographical references and index.
  ISBN 0–8385–0174–5 (case : alk. paper)
  1. Nursing. 2. Community health nursing. I. Burrell, Lenette
  Owens. II. Gerlach, Mary Jo. III. Pless, Betsy S. IV. Adult
  nursing in hospital and community settings.
  [DNLM: 1. Nursing Care. 2. Community Health Nursing. WY 100
  A2444 1996]
  RT41.A354 1996
  610.73—dc20
  DNLM/DLC
  for Library of Congress   96–12365
                                                          CIP

Editor-in-Chief, Nursing: Sally J. Barhydt
Associate Editor: Kathleen L. Riedell
Book Manufacturing Buyer: Anne Armeny
Production Supervisor: Karen Davis
Production Assistants: Jeanmarie Roche, Lisa Guidone
Copy Editor: Genevieve Scandone
Indexer: Maria L. Coughlin
Artist: Gretchen Place
Designer: Janice Barsevich Bielawa
Compositor: Pine Tree Composition
Prepress: Kim Hansen, Jay's Publishers Services
Printer: Courier Kendallville
Cover Art: Lamar Dodd (See frontispiece)

PRINTED IN THE UNITED STATES OF AMERICA

ISBN 0-8385-0174-5

9 780838 501740 90000

VI

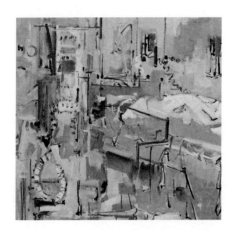

NURSING MANAGEMENT OF ADULTS WITH URINARY PROBLEMS

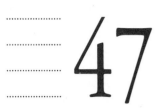

47

Nursing Assessment & Common Urinary Interventions

Kathy Pike Parker and Christine Berding

CHAPTER CONTENTS

■ ASSESSMENT

The major function of the urinary system is to regulate the composition and volume of body fluids. The kidneys have a major role in this process by performing a variety of excretory, metabolic, and regulatory processes that depend on the normal and interrelated functioning of the cardiovascular, nervous, and endocrine systems. Because of the complex nature of these functions, the kidneys are often referred to as "the master chemists of the body."

ANATOMY AND PHYSIOLOGY OVERVIEW

The urinary tract is composed of two kidneys, two ureters, a urinary bladder, and a urethra. Figure 47–1 illustrates the position of these structures in relation to other body structures.

The Kidneys

Functions. The major functions of the kidneys are:

1. To regulate the ionic composition and volume of body fluids and remove metabolic wastes from the blood in the form of urine

2. To assist in controlling the acid–base balance
3. To produce erythropoietin, a hormone that aids in regulating red blood cell production
4. To assist in regulating fluid volume and blood pressure
5. To produce the active form of vitamin D
6. To eliminate drugs and toxic substances
7. To degrade and catabolize peptide hormones

Gross Anatomic Structure. The kidneys are a pair of bean-shaped organs that lie beneath the diaphragm on either side of the vertebral column extending from the twelfth thoracic to the third lumbar vertebra. The kidneys lie against the posterior wall of the abdominal cavity external to the peritoneal lining, so their placement is described as retroperitoneal. Each kidney is approximately 10 to 12 cm (4 to 5 in.) in length, 5.0 to 7.5 cm (2 to 2½ in.) wide, and 2.5 cm (1 in.) thick. Usually, the right kidney is about 1.5 cm lower than the left because of the large area occupied by the liver. Together the kidneys weigh about 300 g (10.6 oz). Each kidney is covered by a tough, fibrous renal capsule and is supported in place by connective tissue called perirenal fat and renal fascia.[69,81] An adrenal gland is located atop each kidney.

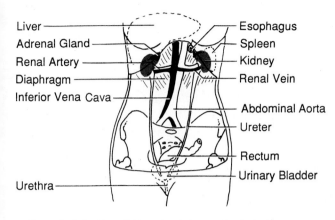

Figure 47–1. Position of kidneys in relation to other body structures.

Macroscopic Structure.

Macroscopic Structure. The kidney can be divided into three major regions: cortex, medulla, and pelvis (Fig. 47–2). The cortex and medulla are the functional renal tissues, whereas the pelvis is part of the collecting system. Collectively, the cortex, medulla, lymphatics, nerves supplying these tissues, and a small amount of connective tissue are called the *renal parenchyma.*

Cortex. The cortex forms the outer portion of the kidney and is approximately 1 cm deep. It lies beneath the renal capsule, surrounds the medulla, and extends downward into the medulla forming renal columns. Because the cortex houses the high-flow vascular portion of the renal functional unit, the *glomerulus,* it receives approximately 90% of renal blood flow at a rate of 4.5 mL/min.

Medulla. The medulla, which is approximately 5 cm deep, contains most of the concentrating portion of the renal functional unit, the tubule system, and is arranged into striated (or striped), fanlike masses called *renal pyramids* (also

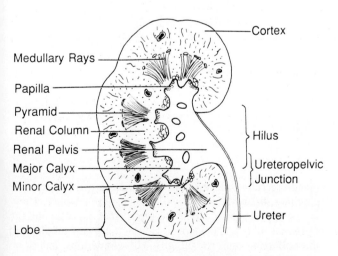

Figure 47–2. Cross section of kidney showing macroscopic structures.

called *medullary rays*). The striated appearance is attributed to the parallel course of the tubules. Each pyramid and its associated cortex form a lobe of the kidney. The medulla receives only approximately 10% of renal blood flow at a rate of 1 mL/min.

Papillae are the terminal tips of the renal pyramids. The papillae have 10 to 25 papillary ducts (called the *ducts of Bellini*) formed by the end fusion of the tubule system. Freshly formed urine is transported through the papillary ducts into a minor calyx, part of the renal pelvis.

Pelvis. The renal pelvis (or sinus) is a funnel-shaped dilation of the upper ureter within the kidney that collects the urine. This cavity has cuplike extensions called *major and minor calyces.* Collectively, the pelvis and calyces can hold approximately 3 to 5 mL of urine. Volumes in excess of this amount may damage the renal tissue. Urine flows through the papillae into the minor calyces, the major calyces, and then into the pelvis. The urine exits the kidney through the ureters, flows into the bladder, and is excreted from the body through the urethra (Fig. 47–1).

Blood, Lymphatic, and Nerve Supply. The hilus (Fig. 47–2) is a longitudinal region located on the concave medial margin of each kidney. Through the hilus pass the major arteries, veins, lymphatics, and nerves that supply the kidney. The *ureteropelvic junction* (Fig. 47–2) refers to the attachment of the upper end of the ureter to the kidney at the hilus.

The kidneys receive approximately 20 to 25% of the cardiac output through the renal arteries, which arise from the abdominal aorta (Fig. 47–1). This portion of the cardiac output is known as the renal fraction and amounts to about 1,200 mL of blood per minute in a 70-kg (150-lb) person. The body's total blood volume circulates through the kidneys about 12 times per hour. Each kidney usually has a single renal artery arising from the aorta that sequentially subdivides into two main segmental (called anterior and posterior branches), then into interlobar, arcuate, and interlobular arteries (Fig. 47–3). The interlobular arteries supply the renal microvascular system (discussed in the next section). The arterial supply of the kidney is vulnerable because the renal artery itself is an end artery, an artery solely responsible for the blood supply of an organ.

The pattern of venous drainage of the kidney corresponds in general to the arterial supply (Fig. 47–3). Blood drains from the renal vein into the inferior vena cava. A rich lymphatic network drains the renal cortex and empties into aortic nodes.

The kidneys receive both sympathetic (adrenergic) and parasympathetic (cholinergic) innervation through nerves that enter at the hilus. The neural supply to the kidneys arises largely from the celiac plexus. The nerves terminate on the walls of blood vessels, where they are believed to have a vasomotor function and on the cells of the urinary tubules.[83] It is important to note that a completely denervated kidney will continue to form urine. When a kidney is transplanted, innervation is interrupted permanently, but renal function remains intact if the transplant is successful.

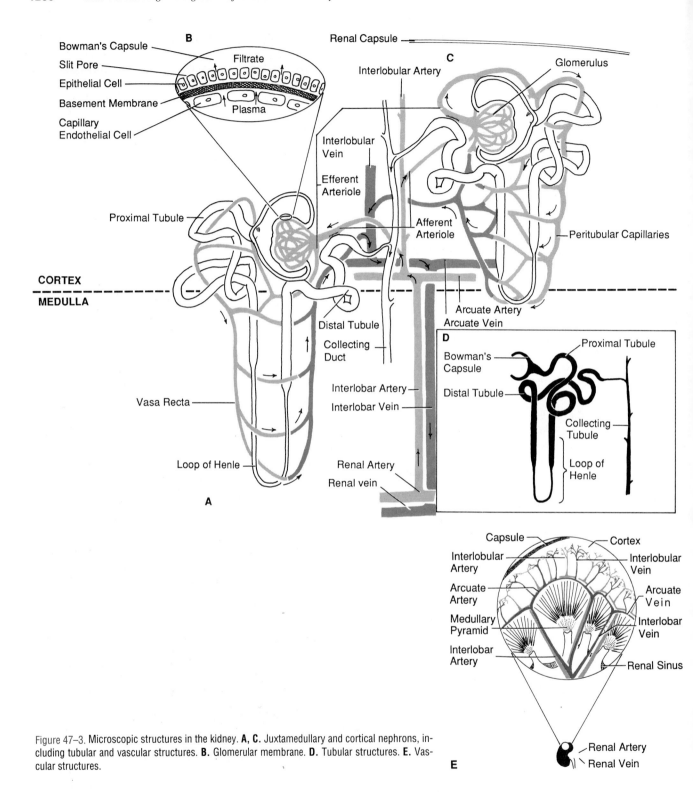

Figure 47–3. Microscopic structures in the kidney. **A, C.** Juxtamedullary and cortical nephrons, including tubular and vascular structures. **B.** Glomerular membrane. **D.** Tubular structures. **E.** Vascular structures.

Microscopic Structure. Each kidney is composed of approximately 1 million microscopic structures called *nephrons* (Fig. 47–3), which are the functional units of the kidney. Each nephron consists of two primary segments—vascular structures and tubular structures (also called the tubule system). The *vascular structures* include the afferent arteriole, the glomerulus, the efferent arteriole, and the peritubular capillary network. The *tubular structures* include Bowman's capsule (also called the glomerular capsule) and the proximal tubule, the loop of Henle, the distal tubule, and the collecting duct (or tubule). The glomerulus and Bowman's capsule together are called the *renal corpuscle* or

Malpighian corpuscle, all of which lie in the cortex of the kidney, along with the proximal and distal tubules. The loop of Henle and the collecting duct dip into the medulla.

Vascular Structures. The afferent arteriole arises from one of the interlobular arteries and supplies blood to the glomerulus, a high-pressure capillary bed. The glomerulus is semipermeable and therefore permits fluid and particles from within the blood (collectively known as the *glomerular filtrate*), to pass into Bowman's capsule. The glomerular capillaries then reunite to form the efferent arteriole. The efferent arteriole divides into a second, low-pressure capillary bed, the *peritubular capillary network.* This low-pressure capillary bed surrounds the tubule system, nourishes it, and permits the exchange of substances between the tubules and the blood. The blood then flows into an interlobular vein.

Usually, arterioles form a single capillary system that drains into venules, but the kidneys have a unique two-capillary structure. The glomeruli function similarly to the arterial ends of the tissue capillaries whereby fluid and solutes leave the capillaries. In contrast, the peritubular capillaries function similarly to the venous ends of the systemic capillaries, with fluid and necessary solutes being reabsorbed from the tubules into the peritubular capillary network.

Tubular Structures. These structures function in conjunction with the vascular structures. *Bowman's capsule* is a cuplike structure that almost completely surrounds the glomerulus (Fig. 47–3) and collects the glomerular filtrate. The remainder of the tubule system is composed of a long, coiled, and looped tube that is attached proximally to Bowman's capsule and emerges distally in the renal papillae.

The *proximal tubule* (also called the *proximal convoluted tubule*) is a short, coiled segment directly connected to Bowman's capsule and located in the cortex of the kidney along with the renal corpuscle. The *loop of Henle,* a hairpinlike structure with descending and ascending limbs, begins at the proximal tubule, dips into the medulla, and rises into the cortex. The wall of the descending limb and the lower end of the ascending limb are very thin and therefore are called the thin segments of the loop of Henle. The upper portion of the ascending limb becomes thick like the other portions of the tubule system and is called the thick segment of the ascending limb.[31,65] The ascending limb of Henle is attached to the coiled *distal tubule* (also called the *distal convoluted tubule*) that lies in the cortex. Finally, the *collecting duct* (also called the *collecting tubule*) straightens and dips into the medulla. The collecting tubules join to form progressively larger ducts and finally drain into the pelvis through the papillary ducts.

Types of Nephrons. Although all nephrons are basically similar, they differ somewhat in structure and function. Approximately 85% of the nephrons are referred to as *cortical nephrons* (Fig. 47–3). They are located in the superficial areas of the cortex and have short loops of Henle that extend superficially into the medulla. These loops of Henle receive their blood supply from the peritubular capillary bed.

The remaining 15% of the nephrons are called the *juxtamedullary nephrons.* The renal corpuscle of these nephrons is located deeper in the cortex. In addition, the loop of Henle is longer and extends deeply into the medulla. The peritubular capillaries of this type of nephron are very specialized and are called the *vasa recta* (Fig. 47–3). The vasa recta are composed of parallel loops of vessels that surround the loop of Henle and have an important role in urine concentration.

Renal Interstitium. This is composed of tissues in the spaces around each tubule—between the tubules and peritubular capillaries in the cortex and between the parallel tubules in the medulla. This tissue consists of interstitial cells, connective tissue, collagen, capillaries, lymphatic vessels, and motor and sensory nerves. These tissues are especially abundant in the medulla.

Urine Formation

Urine is formed by three processes: glomerular filtration, tubular reabsorption, and tubular secretion.

Glomerular Filtration. This is the passage of fluid and other substances from the blood in the glomerulus, through the glomerular membrane, and into Bowman's capsule as a result of a pressure differential. Because of the special structure of the membrane of the glomerular capillaries (Fig. 47–3B), it is highly permeable to solvent (fluid) and solutes (particles).

The glomerular membrane has three major layers. The endothelial cells line the glomerulus and are perforated by thousands of microscopic holes called *fenestrae.* Outside this layer is a basement membrane composed of collagen and glycoproteins. The collagen provides structural strength, and the negatively charged glycoproteins discourage filtration of plasma proteins. The final layer of the epithelial cells, which is actually the inner layer of Bowman's capsule, line the outside of the glomerulus. These cells are not continuous but instead are formed by fingerlike projections called *podocytes* that cover the outer surface of the basement membrane. Because of the small pore size (slit pores), this complex microscopic structure prevents many substances from passing through, including blood cells and proteins. An exception is albumin, which has a low molecular weight and passes into the filtrate in small quantities. Most of the albumin is subsequently reabsorbed by the proximal tubules, so only small amounts (less than 20 mg/24 hr) pass into the urine.[65] Thus, except for blood cells, protein, and insignificant amounts of albumin, glomerular filtrate is composed of the same substances as normal plasma, including glucose, vitamins, minerals, amino acids, sodium, chloride, potassium, and other electrolytes.

Glomerular Filtration Rate. The amount of glomerular filtrate formed per minute is called the glomerular filtration rate (GFR). In the normal person, the GFR is approximately 90 to 125 mL/min or about 180 L/day. The kidneys receive 20 to 25% of the cardiac output or over 1,500 L/day of blood. As approximately 45% of that volume is cells, the remaining volume is referred to as *renal plasma*. The portion of the renal plasma flow that becomes glomerular filtrate is called the *filtration fraction*. The renal plasma flow is approximately 650 mL/min and the GFR is 125 mL/min, and so the filtration fraction is approximately 19%. Over 99% of this filtrate is reabsorbed by the tubule system, with the remaining fluid flowing into the renal pelvis as urine. Thus, normal urinary output is approximately 1.25 mL/min, 75 mL/hr, or 1,800 mL/day.

The GFR is determined by three primary forces: hydrostatic pressure of blood in the glomerulus, colloid osmotic pressure of the blood, and hydrostatic pressure of Bowman's capsule. Hydrostatic pressure of the blood is the pressure exerted against the walls of a vessel by the force of the blood within the walls. The major control of the pressure within the glomerulus is maintained by changes in the degree of constriction of the afferent and efferent arterioles, a process called *autoregulation*. Increased constriction of the afferent arteriole decreases the blood flow and pressure in the glomerulus and causes a subsequent decrease in GFR. Conversely, constriction of the efferent arteriole increases the pressure in the glomerulus and increases GFR. The average pressure in the glomerulus is approximately 55 to 70 mm Hg.

Colloid osmotic pressure of the blood is maintained by the proteins and is a "pulling in" force as opposed to the "pushing out" force of hydrostatic pressure. The lower the colloid osmotic pressure, as with a patient with hypoproteinemia, the higher the GFR. On the other hand, a patient with hyperproteinemia would tend to have a lower GFR.

As Bowman's capsule almost completely surrounds the glomerulus, it normally exerts a small hydrostatic pressure against glomerular filtration, which is estimated to be about 18 mm Hg. In urinary obstruction or severe inflammation with edema, this pressure increases considerably. If the hydrostatic pressure of Bowman's capsule exceeds the hydrostatic pressure of the blood in the glomerulus, glomerular filtration will cease. These and other factors that influence the GFR are listed in Table 47–1.

The GFR may be summarized by the following equation:

$$GFR = HP(b) - COP(b) - HP(BC)$$

Glomular filtration rate (GFR) equals hydrostatic pressure in the glomerular blood (HP[b]) minus colloid osmotic pressure in the glomerular blood (COP[b]) minus hydrostatic pressure in Bowman's capsule (HP[BC]).

Tubular Reabsorption and Secretion. When the glomerular filtrate enters the tubule from Bowman's capsule, it contains many valuable constituents, including important electrolytes and water. As the glomerular filtrate passes through the tubules, its volume is reduced and its composition altered by *tubular reabsorption*, a process that occurs through active transport, diffusion, and osmosis. In this process, water and solutes are reabsorbed from the tubular fluid into

---

TABLE 47–1

FACTORS AFFECTING THE GLOMERULAR FILTRATION RATE

1. Changes in renal blood flow
2. Changes in glomerular capillary hydrostatic pressure
   a. Changes in systemic blood pressure
   b. Afferent or efferent arteriolar constriction
3. Changes in hydrostatic pressure in Bowman's capsule
   a. Ureteral obstruction
   b. Edema of kidney inside tight renal capsule
4. Changes in concentration of plasma proteins: dehydration, hypoproteinemia
5. Changes in glomerular filter
   a. Changes in capillary permeability
   b. Changes in surface area

(Source: *Ganong*.[28])

---

the interstitial spaces, then into the peritubular capillaries. Thus, the important constituents are returned to the bloodstream. Substances such as glucose, amino acids, and vitamins are normally completely reabsorbed and do not appear in the urine.

Tubular secretion is the process by which some substances are secreted from the blood into the tubular lumen of the nephron. Tubular secretion is very important in regulating potassium and hydrogen ion concentrations. In addition, a number of drugs, such as penicillin, are removed from the blood, primarily by active secretion rather than by glomerular filtration.

In some cases both processes—reabsorption and secretion—work together to permit the flexible regulation of a given substance. Large amounts of filtered sodium, chloride, calcium, magnesium, and phosphate are reabsorbed. Only small amounts of these substances are secreted, with the quantity varying according to the dietary intake of these solutes and the body's metabolic requirements.

Proximal Tubule. As previously mentioned, the GFR is approximately 125 mL/min. As this fluid passes into the proximal tubule, about 65% of the sodium content is actively reabsorbed, along with the obligatory reabsorption of 65% (or 80 mL) of the water. Thus, only 45 mL/min of an isotonic filtrate flows into the loop of Henle.[65] Other substances that are reabsorbed are listed in Table 47–2. It is important to note that the proximal tubule is essential in the reabsorption of glucose. In the normal individual, all glucose is reabsorbed. The normal renal glucose threshold is approximately 300 mg/dL, but this can vary greatly.[66]

Loop of Henle. The isotonic filtrate then passes into the thin descending loop of Henle, which is highly permeable to

TABLE 47-2

RENAL HANDLING OF VARIOUS PLASMA CONSTITUENTS IN A NORMAL ADULT HUMAN ON AN AVERAGE DIET

Substance	Per 24 Hours				Percentage Reabsorbed	Location[a]
	Filtered	*Reabsorbed*	*Secreted*	*Excreted*		
Na⁺ (mEq)	26,000	25,850		150	99.4	P, L, D, C
K⁺ (mEq)	600	560[b]	50[b]	90	93.3	P, L, D, C
Cl⁻ (mEq)	18,000	17,850		150	99.2	P, L, D, C
HCO₃⁻ (mEq)	4,900	4,900		0	100	P, D
Urea (mmol)	870	460[c]		410	53	P, L, D, C
Creatinine (mmol)	12	1[d]	1[d]	12	—	—
Uric acid (mmol)	50	49	4	5	98	P
Glucose (mmol)	800	800		0	100	P
Total solute (mOsm)	54,000	53,400	100	700	87	P, L, D, C
Water (mL)	180,000	179,000		1,000	99.4	P, L, D, C

[a]P, proximal tubules; L, loops of Henle; D, distal tubules; C, collecting ducts.
[b]K⁺ is both reabsorbed and secreted.
[c]Urea diffuses into as well as out of some portions of the nephron.
[d]Variable secretion and probable reabsorption of creatinine in humans.
(Source: *Ganong.*[28])

water but only minimally permeable to urea, sodium, and other ions (Fig. 47–4). Approximately 15 to 20% of the filtrate is reabsorbed. As the filtrate passes into the ascending limb, which is characterized by low permeability to water and high permeability to sodium and chloride; sodium and chloride passively diffuse into the interstitium. Although small amounts of the sodium and chloride may passively diffuse back into the descending limb, most remain within

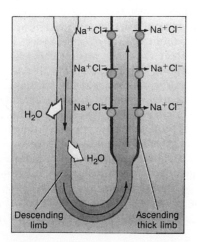

Figure 47–4. Movement of water, sodium, and chloride along the loop of Henle. (*From Martini.*[46])

the interstitium and help maintain medullary hypertonicity. The normal serum osmolality is 285 to 295 mOsm/L, whereas the osmolality of the medulla increases from approximately 300 mOsm/L in its outer region to about 1,200 mOsm/L in its inner region. The maintenance of this hypertonicity is important in urine concentration. The process by which it is maintained is referred to as the *countercurrent multiplication mechanism.*

As the filtrate passes into the thick ascending limb, additional sodium and chloride are actively absorbed, causing the filtrate to become relatively hypotonic. The net effect of the passage of the approximately 45 mL/min of filtrate through the loop of Henle is that approximately 25 mL/min of a dilute filtrate passes into the distal tubules. This represents 20% of the original amount of glomerular filtrate.

Distal Tubule. This tubule, particularly its first part, is relatively impermeable to water.[28] However, the reabsorption of sodium and potassium is regulated by aldosterone, a mineralocorticoid produced by the adrenal cortex. Depending on the body's needs, hydrogen and bicarbonate ions are also either secreted or reabsorbed in the distal tubule, and ammonium ions are secreted.

Collecting Tubule. This tubule is the final site of concentration or dilution of urine and receives about 9.3% of the original amount of glomerular filtrate or approximately 12 mL/min. The fluid reabsorption is controlled by antidiuretic hormone

(ADH), which is secreted by the posterior pituitary. The presence of ADH causes the collecting tubule to become highly permeable to water, permitting the absorption of water into the medulla, and thus making the urine more concentrated.[28]

Renal Regulatory Mechanisms

The kidneys have major roles in the regulation of water, electrolytes, and acid–base balance and in excretion of metabolites.

Renal Regulation of Water.
The largest constituent of the human body is water. In healthy, lean adults, water constitutes 55 to 65% of the total body weight. In females and the elderly, the proportion of water is slightly less, most likely because the ratio of muscle to water-poor tissues, such as fat and bone, is lower.[81] Approximately 55 to 75% of this total body water is intracellular, or inside the cells; about one third to one half of this fluid is tightly bound to cartilage and/or bone and is relatively inaccessible. The remainder of the body fluid is extracellular, being divided into the (1) intravascular fluid (plasma) and (2) the extravascular fluid (interstitial). The equilibrium of fluid between the extracellular and intracellular compartments is maintained because most of the membranes that separate these compartments are freely permeable to water. Thus, this water is described as *free water.*

The renal handling of free water is regulated primarily by ADH, also called *vasopressin,* which is produced by the hypothalamus and stored in the posterior pituitary. Several variables that affect the secretion of ADH include plasma osmolality (probably the most important), blood volume, blood pressure, and gain or loss of fluids.[81]

The release of ADH is mediated by neurons called *osmoreceptors* located in the hypothalamus. These osmoreceptors trigger the production of ADH when the osmolality reaches a certain threshold level. Above this threshold, ADH is released in direct proportion to the plasma osmolality. Below this threshold, ADH production is suppressed. The thirst mechanism also provides an important adjunct to the ADH control of water balance. In healthy adults, a rise in plasma osmolality of only 2 to 3% produces the desire to drink; however, the level at which thirst is stimulated varies significantly from person to person. In addition, some drugs and hormones (high doses of morphine, isoproterenol, epinephrine, and insulin) can stimulate ADH production, whereas others (norepinephrine, low doses of morphine, and alcohol) can inhibit ADH production. Thus, these drugs and hormones may have a significant role in free water regulation in pathophysiologic conditions.[81]

The renal conservation or excretion of free water is determined primarily by the presence or absence of ADH, which controls the permeability of the collecting tubules to water. When ADH is absent, these tubules are almost entirely impermeable to water so that water is excreted. When ADH is present, the collecting tubules become highly permeable to water so that water is reabsorbed into the vascular system.

Renal Regulation of Electrolytes.
The kidneys assist in the regulation of many electrolytes. The renal handling of sodium and potassium is discussed because these are very important *cations* (positively charged electrolytes). Sodium is the dominant extracellular cation, whereas potassium is the dominant intracellular cation.

Sodium. The major factors that affect the renal handling of sodium include (1) the renal blood flow, (2) the glomerular filtration rate, (3) the tubular concentration of sodium and flow of filtrate, and (4) the presence or absence of several hormones, including aldosterone. In states of *hypoperfusion* when renal blood flow, glomerular filtrate, and tubular flow are decreased, the concentration of sodium within the tubular lumen is increased. Some sodium is reabsorbed because it is needed by the body. In states of *hyperperfusion,* such as osmotic diuresis or increased water intake, both salt and water reabsorption are restricted.[81]

Aldosterone is released in response to both hyponatremic and hyperkalemic states. Aldosterone release increases the reabsorption of sodium and the excretion of potassium in the distal and collecting tubules.

Atrial natriuretic hormone (ANH) is released by the heart in response to increased right atrial pressure. ANH stimulates an increase in GFR and inhibition of sodium and water recovery in the distal nephron. It therefore is important in both sodium and water balance.[51]

Potassium. The major factors that affect the renal handling of potassium include potassium intake, acid–base balance, and aldosterone. An increase in the dietary intake of potassium is normally followed by a corresponding increase in potassium secretion by the distal tubule. Thus, in the presence of normal renal function, it is virtually impossible to ingest too much potassium; however, in renal insufficiency or failure, this mechanism is seriously impaired, leading to the possibility of developing dangerously high serum potassium levels.

A change in extracellular hydrogen ion concentration, or pH, also affects renal handling of potassium. Metabolic and respiratory alkalosis stimulates the renal excretion of potassium, whereas metabolic and respiratory acidosis depresses the renal excretion of potassium.

Aldosterone directly affects the distal and collecting tubules to promote the active reabsorption of sodium from the tubules and active secretion of potassium into the tubules. *Hyperkalemia* stimulates the adrenal cortex to increase aldosterone production, which causes an increase in the renal secretion of potassium. In *hypokalemia,* aldosterone production decreases with a corresponding decrease in potassium excretion. Other factors that increase potassium excretion include excess mineralocorticoid production and potassium-losing diuretics such as chlorothiazide, furosemide, and mannitol. Factors that decrease potassium excretion include adrenal mineralocorticoid deficiency and potassium-sparing diuretics such as spironolactone.

Renal Regulation of Acid–Base Balance.
Without the body's buffering mechanisms, body fluids would become increas-

Innervation (Fig. 47–7) of the bladder is complex. The bladder is the only part of the urinary tract that is totally dependent on intact innervation to serve its functions.[80] Nerves supplying the bladder form the vesical plexus, which arises from the third to fourth sacral segments of the spinal cord. The plexus contains sympathetic and parasympathetic nerve fibers and sensory (afferent) fibers. The motor (efferent) innervation of the bladder is contained within the sympathetic and parasympathetic nerve fibers. The efferent parasympathetic fibers distribute motor fibers to the detrusor muscle and inhibitory fibers to the internal urethral sphincter.

The sympathetic nerves to the bladder have no part in micturition. They do mediate the contraction of the male internal urethral sphincter that prevents reflux of semen into the bladder during ejaculation.[28]

In the resting state, the bladder is in a state of sympathetic tone with the detrusor relaxed and the internal sphincter closed. Normal filling and emptying of the bladder are controlled by the parasympathetic nervous system. With the urge to urinate, the sympathetic tone is inhibited and the parasympathetic fibers are stimulated; this causes contraction of the detrusor and inhibition (relaxation) of the internal sphincter.

The external urethral sphincter, supplied by the pudendal nerve, is also concerned with controlling micturition. The sensory nerves of the bladder are concerned with either pain or the conscious awareness of bladder distention.

Intrinsic tension of the skeletal muscular ring surrounding the neck of the bladder and the adjacent proximal urethra prevents the urine from continuously leaking. Contraction of the detrusor muscle during voiding widens this ring, allowing urine to escape through the urethra. Bladder emptying is a very efficient process. If bladder function is normal, there is from 25 to 50 mL of residual urine (urine remaining in the bladder after voiding).

Micturition. When the bladder has reached a capacity of about 200 mL, the urge to urinate begins. The adult bladder normally has a capacity of 350 to 450 mL.[80] Micturition (the act of urinating or voiding) commonly takes place when the bladder contains about 280 mL of urine. Although the bladder can tolerate about 500 mL, discomfort is experienced at levels above this amount because of the tension on the bladder wall. When the bladder is distended to an average degree, it measures about 5 cm (2 in.) in height. In excessive distention, it may extend as far as the umbilicus or even higher. The act of micturition involves the coordinated contraction of the detrusor muscle, muscles of the pelvic floor, and relaxation of the internal and external urethral sphincters.

Micturition Reflex and Termination of Urination. When the bladder fills, tension in its wall causes impulses to be sent along pelvic nerves to the spinal cord to the spinal center for micturition, and also up the spinal cord to the brain stem micturition reflex center and the voluntary control micturition center in the cerebral cortex. During the first feeling of an urge to void, the spinal center is inhibited by the brain stem center. As the bladder expands and tension increases, pain results and it is necessary for the cerebral cortex voluntary center to inhibit the spinal center.

Once a suitable place for voiding is found, this voluntary control is lifted and the spinal center discharges parasympathetic impulses, which cause detrusor contraction and opening of the urethra. The voluntary center can also force the spinal reflex center inhibition to be lifted in the case of low urine volume (which allows one to urinate when there is no urge). Once a voiding contraction occurs, it is maintained by impulses from the brain stem center (which can be overridden by the voluntary cerebral center, allowing one to stop in midstream), until the bladder is emptied and there is no tension stimulus.

The Urethra

The urethra is the tube that extends from the base of the bladder to an external opening called the *meatus* through which urine is expelled from the bladder. Differences in the male and female urethra are illustrated in Chaps. 62 and 64.

Male Urethra. The male urethra measures from 18 to 20 cm (7 to 8 in.) long. The reproductive and urinary systems share this outlet from the body. Because the prostate gland is located below the bladder neck and surrounds the urethra completely, when enlarged, it can cause major difficulties in the functioning of the urinary tract.

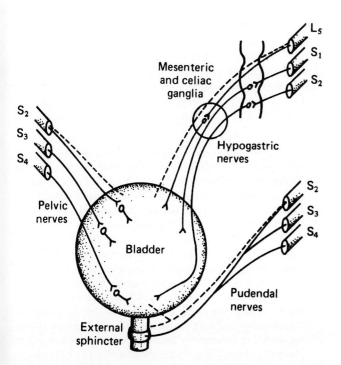

Figure 47–7. Innervation of the bladder. Dashed lines indicate sensory nerves. Parasympathetic innervation is shown at left, sympathetic at upper right, and somatic at lower right. (*From Ganong.*[28])

The urethra is divided into three connected sections.

1. The *prostatic section,* about 3 cm long, extends through the prostate gland. The ejaculating ducts of the reproductive system empty into the proximal end. This is the widest part of the urethra.

2. The *membranous section,* about 1 to 2 cm long, is the shortest, least dilatable, and narrowest section.

3. The *spongy cavernous* (or *penile*) *section* is about 15 cm (6 in.) long. Located in the bulb of the penis, it extends to the meatus on the tip of the penis.

The urethra is composed of mucous membrane that is continuous internally with that of the bladder; submucous tissue that consists of a vascular, erectile layer; and a layer of smooth and voluntary muscle.

Female Urethra. The female urethra is about 4 cm (1½ in.) long and 6 mm in diameter. It is slightly curved and lies beneath the symphysis pubis just anterior to the vagina.[79] The urethral meatus is located in the vaginal vestibule about 2.5 cm (1 in.) behind the clitoris.

Like the male urethra, the female urethra contains muscular, erectile, and mucous layers in its wall. The muscular layer is continuous with the muscular layer of the bladder and extends the entire length of the tube. A thin layer of erectile tissue containing a plexus of large veins, muscle fibers, and connective tissue lies underneath the mucous coat. The mucous membrane continues externally with the mucous membrane of the vulva and internally with the bladder.

PATHOPHYSIOLOGY OVERVIEW

Table 47–3 correlates the major structures and their functions with the terms and their definitions of the major pathophysiology. Each disorder is discussed in the forthcoming chapters in this section.

HISTORY AND PHYSICAL EXAMINATION
Psychosocial Implications

In most societies, voiding is an activity done in private. This is especially true for females, in that voiding requires removing undergarments. The process of voiding is not discussed in social settings and because of this cultural set, many individuals are uncomfortable discussing personal habits and irregularities related to the urinary tract.

Nurses need to be aware of this awkwardness when obtaining the history, requesting individuals to provide urine samples, or especially when performing a urinary catheterization or other invasive procedure. Privacy is needed for both discussion of the urinary tract and sample collection. Patients may be more likely to experience embarrassment if they have not had any previous difficulties with their urinary tract. Having a stranger, sometimes of the opposite sex, expose or discuss the perineal area may also be a great cause for concern. Therefore, every effort must be made to help the person feel at ease.

It is appropriate to display a professional manner and use correct terminology; however, when talking with individuals who have urinary problems, it may be necessary to use various colloquial terms that refer to the act of voiding. Factors to consider in choosing terms include the patient's age, educational level, and sociocultural state. Terms that may be used include "pee," "pee-pee." "tee-tee," "take a leak," "make water," "pass water," "#l," and "relieve oneself."

Disorders of the urinary tract are often associated with considerable pain or discomfort, particularly when voiding. When this is the case, the patient should be supported and made as comfortable as possible during the history taking and collection of the urine specimen.

History
Chief Complaint and History of the Present Illness. Signs and symptoms (or clinical findings) that prompt the individual to seek help are usually related to variations in the voiding pattern, pain, and changes in urine. It is important to determine when symptoms were first noticed, precipitating factors, and the setting surrounding the problem (such as specific activities or conditions associated with their onset), the general pattern of the illness episode (such as acute or slow onset, or intermittent symptoms), and whether the individual has ever experienced a similar episode. It is important to know what has been done to treat the problem. Some patients may take medications they have at home that will alter the culture and sensitivity of the urine.

Variations in the Voiding Patterns. Many urinary tract disorders are manifested by variations in urination (also called *voiding* or *micturition*). The amount of urinary output is an accessible monitor of therapeutic progress. Because voiding occurs several times each day, the patient can readily describe the voiding pattern and may be quick to notice changes in the appearance or odor of the urine. However, changes in voiding patterns often occur gradually and sometimes without accompanying pain, and so the patient may have accepted certain changes as normal and forget to mention them without prompting. The following factors can be used to guide the assessment of alterations in voiding.

1. *Number of times that urination occurs per day (urinary frequency).* An increase may be caused by decreased bladder capacity from inflammation, infection, neurogenic disorders, presence of a foreign body, or a chemical or radiation injury. Frequency may also occur when the bladder is distended for a long period, as with almost complete obstruction (distention with overflow).

2. *Number of times an individual arises to void at night (nocturia) and the approximate volume.* This can be caused by the same problems as mentioned above, plus the mobilization of fluid in dependent edema or the poorly timed ingestion of diuretics (such as late afternoon or night). In addition, nocturia may be the first sign of renal insufficiency and may indicate that the kidneys are losing the ability to concentrate the urine. It is most commonly a symptom of an enlarged prostate in men.

3. *Inability to void or difficulty voiding* (difficulty starting the stream—called *hesitancy*). This may signal an obstructive disorder in the lower urinary tract or a neurologic disorder.

TABLE 47–3

OVERVIEW OF ANATOMY, PHYSIOLOGY, AND RELATED PATHOPHYSIOLOGY OF THE URINARY SYSTEM

Anatomy and Physiology	Pathophysiology
Kidney	
Glomeruli: Clusters of capillaries that filter the blood and produce *glomerular filtrate,* composed of the same substances as plasma, without significant amounts of protein and no blood cells. Glomerular filtrate is the first step in urine formation.	*Glomerulopathies:* General term describing a host of diseases characterized by pathologic changes of the glomerulus; frequently divided into primary and secondary types. *Primary glomerular diseases* are thought to be caused by immunologic mechanisms; they include acute glomerulonephritis and nephrotic syndrome. *Secondary glomerular diseases* occur secondary to an overall disease process such as infection, collagen vascular disease, or exposure to toxins.
Glomerular filtrate normally contains no significant amount of protein.	*Proteinuria:* An altered glomerular capillary wall allows protein to enter glomerular filtrate; may be caused by various disorders.
Nephrotic syndrome: Excessive proteinuria, leading to hypoproteinuria.
Multiple myeloma: Produces proteinuria from production of excessive immunoglobin lightchains.
Glomerular filtrate normally contains no red blood cells or white blood cells.	*Hematuria:* Presence of red blood cells in the urine; commonly seen in urinary tract infections and stone disease.
Pyuria: Presence of white blood cells; seen in urinary tract infection and stone disease.
Tubules: Major site for renal regulation of water, electrolytes, and acid–base balance.	*Electrolyte abnormalities* resulting from kidney dysfunction are described below.
Tubules are the major site for regulation of water balance as they concentrate or dilute the urine.	Tubular disorders may affect the kidney's ability to excrete or reabsorb water. In early stages of *acute* renal failure, tubular destruction frequently results in *oliguria* (100 to 500 mL daily urine output) or *anuria* (< 100 mL daily urine output). In early stages of *chronic* renal failure, large amounts of dilute urine may be produced because of the diminishing ability of tubules to concentrate the urine.
Tubules are the major site for regulation of potassium.	Disorders of potassium imbalance may result from tubular disorders.
Hyperkalemia: From decreased excretory mechanisms of tubule; common in renal failure.
Hypokalemia: From increased excretory mechanisms of tubule.
Large amounts of filtered sodium are reabsorbed by the tubules.	Sodium imbalance may occur. *Hyponatremia:* Sodium loss or sodium depletion may be caused by renal tubular disease.
Tubules are the site for regulation of acid–base balance. The primary renal mechanism involved in acid–base control is tubular secretion of hydrogen.	*Metabolic acidosis* may develop because of excessive body content of nonvolatile acids and a decrease in concentration of plasma bicarbonate.
Kidneys normally receive 25% of cardiac output.	Hypotension, dehydration, and cardiogenic shock may lead to decreased blood flow to the kidneys; *prerenal failure* may result. If volume or blood pressure is corrected promptly, normal renal function usually returns. If ischemia continues, *intrarenal failure* (also called *acute tubular necrosis*) develops.
Although plasma glucose is freely filterable across the glomerulus, it is normally entirely reabsorbed in the proximal tubules; therefore, urine normally contains no glucose.	*Glycosuria* (glucose in the urine) is most commonly seen in diabetes mellitus, when serum glucose may exceed the reabsorptive capacity (or threshold) of the proximal tubule; however, disorders of the proximal tubule may also permit glucose to "spill" into the urine, even in the presence of a normal serum glucose level.
Although urea is reabsorbed by the renal tubules to some extent, it is excreted in high concentrations.	By-products of metabolism may be retained and produce *azotemia* (retention of urea and other metabolites), especially with renal insufficiency.
The majority of uric acid is reabsorbed along the tubular pathway.	*Hyperuricemia* (excessive accumulation of uric acid) results when tubules are unable to excrete uric acid.

(Continued)

TABLE 47-3   *(Continued)*

OVERVIEW OF ANATOMY, PHYSIOLOGY, AND RELATED PATHOPHYSIOLOGY OF THE URINARY SYSTEM

Anatomy and Physiology	Pathophysiology
Kidneys produce and release erythropoietin, which stimulates red blood cell production.	Loss of functional renal tissue is associated with *anemia* related to decreased production of erythropoietin.
Kidneys convert vitamin D to 1,25-DHCC, a hormone that promotes intestinal absorption of calcium.	Loss of functional renal tissue leads to decreased ability to convert vitamin D to 1,25-DHCC, resulting in hypocalcemia.
Nephrons are important in the degradation of gastrin, a hormone secreted by stomach mucosa that stimulates production of hydrochloric acid.	In renal failure, gastrin is not adequately degraded, so higher levels remain in the body and may contribute to gastric irritation and bleeding.
The *juxtaglomerular apparatus* in the kidney produces the hormone *renin,* which elevates the blood pressure.	Increased secretion of renin can lead to hypertension.
The kidneys normally degrade about 20% of the insulin secreted by the pancreas.	The decreased ability of the kidneys to degrade insulin may lead to higher circulating levels. The insulin requirement usually decreases significantly in the diabetic patient who develops renal failure.
Ureters	
Paired muscular tubes that transport urine from the renal pelvis to the bladder.	Obstruction (commonly from urinary calculi) may cause a *hydroureter* above obstruction; also causes reflux of urine into the kidney pelvis.
Bladder	
Muscular storage vessel for urine.	Bladder musculature may be altered as a result of *urinary obstruction.* In the *compensation stage,* smooth muscle in the bladder hypertrophies and intravesicular pressure is increased to overcome outlet resistance.
	In the *decompensation stage,* bladder tone is impaired; the contraction phase is too short to expel urine *completely.*
	Uninhibited bladder contractions result in *urgency incontinence,* and *incomplete emptying.*
	Diverticuli (saclike outpouchings) may be produced when mucosa is forced through musculature of the bladder wall.
Urethra	
Tubular passageway for urine to be excreted; sphincter controls urination.	*Hypotonic internal sphincter* results in urinary incontinence when urine meets no resistance. If the urethral sphincter and bladder do not work harmoniously, *sphincter dyssynergia* caused by a *hypotonic internal sphincter* can develop.
	Hypertonic internal sphincter results in urinary retention as flow of urine is obstructed.
External urethral sphincter (in males only): Assists in controlling urination.	With a *hypotonic external sphincter,* urine meets no resistance and urinary incontinence occurs.
	With a *hypertonic external sphincter,* flow of urine is obstructed and urinary retention occurs.

4. *Burning or discomfort on voiding (dysuria) with associated suprapubic aching or spasms; also, sudden strong desire to void (urgency) that may occur soon after having voided.* This is usually a sign of infection in the bladder or urethra, but may be related to calculi (stones), nonbacterial inflammations, foreign bodies, tumors, or prostatitis.

5. *Estimated urinary output.* An unusually low urinary output (oliguria [100 to 500 mL urine in 24 hours] or *anuria* [less than 100 mL in 24 hours]) may indicate renal insuffi-

ciency or may be caused by hypovolemia, shock, trauma, an incompatible blood transfusion, or drug toxicity. An unusually large urine volume (*polyuria*) occurs in diabetes mellitus, diabetes insipidus, some types of chronic renal failure, and ingestion of diuretics.

6. *Involuntary voiding (incontinence).*
   • *Enuresis* is incontinence that occurs during sleep. It may be related to a psychogenic disorder, obstruction, infection, or a neurogenic dysfunction.

- *Stress incontinence* occurs with physical strain, such as coughing or sneezing. It is usually related to pelvic relaxation after childbirth.
- *Dribbling* or "dripping urine" is overflow incontinence, which indicates that the weakened or overdistended bladder cannot contract to generate a stream of urine or there is prostatic obstruction.
- *Continuous urinary leakage* refers to total incontinence. It may be related to damage to the external sphincter or adjacent structures, including a vesicovaginal fistula, neurogenic conditions, or structural anomalies.

Pain. Although pain does not always accompany urinary disorders, when it is present the patient almost always comes to the health care system for relief. The specific location and degree of pain vary greatly according to the organ involved and the cause of the pain. The pain may be local or referred to another area. Distention within the urinary tract is the most common cause, but inflammation and foreign bodies may also produce pain.

- *Kidney pain* may be caused by diseased kidneys. It may produce a dull pain in the back and in the *costovertebral angle* (CVA) area (angle between the lower ribs and adjacent vertebrae; Fig. 47–8) and spread toward the umbilicus.
- *Renal or ureteral colic* is usually described as severe, sharp, stabbing, and excruciating; it may radiate from the kidney to the bladder and urethra and is sometimes felt in the flank (area between the ribs and upper border of ilium), testes, or ovaries (Fig. 47–8).
- *Bladder pain* is often described as a dull, continuous suprapubic discomfort. It is usually associated with infection and bladder distention. Sharp, intermittent pain may indicate spasm of the bladder, which is also associated with infection.
- *Urethral pain* is usually associated with inflammation or presence of a foreign body. A burning sensation on voiding that may be followed by spasmlike pain is produced by inflammation.
- *Prostatic pain* is usually associated with acute prostatitis and described as a vague discomfort or full feeling in the perineal or rectal areas. If acute obstruction occurs, bladder pain and backache may occur.

Changes in the Urine. Ask the patient if any changes have been noticed in the appearance or odor of the urine. Many patients with urinary complaints will have noticed gross hematuria, although sometimes the hematuria is microscopic. Ask when the red color was first noticed and establish related circumstances when possible. Ask whether blood was observed on the toilet tissue after voiding. When hematuria is reported, pursue possible systemic causes by asking about the ingestion of anticoagulants, such as coumarin, antiplatelet drugs such as aspirin, or medications that are known to color urine red, such as Pyridium.

The urine may transiently become a dark "cola" color associated with severe physical stress, exercise, or trauma. This may be related to the release of large amounts of myoglobin from damaged muscle, which filters into the urine. The dark urine color may be present for only a few hours, but it is diagnostically extremely important. Ask if a foul odor or a cloudy white appearance to the urine has been noticed, which suggests a urinary tract infection.

Additional Clinical Findings. Because the urinary organs are adjacent to and share autonomic and sensory innervations with the gastrointestinal (GI) system, GI complaints often accompany urinary complaints. Ask specifically about nausea, vomiting, anorexia, diarrhea, abdominal discomfort, and other GI manifestations. Generalized itching or irritation of the skin may occur from increased toxic substances on the skin when the kidneys are unable to remove waste products normally. Likewise, edema is commonly observed when the kidney is unable to remove excess body fluid.

Ask about secretions or drainage from the urinary meatus. Because of the proximity of the urinary and genital tracts, female patients with urinary complaints should also be questioned about (1) drainage from the genital tract, as may occur with fungus infections or some sexually transmitted diseases and (2) current menstruation because erythrocytes may be present in the urinalysis from this source if the specimen is not collected carefully.

Finally, listen for general complaints such as malaise, fever, and weight loss. These may indicate an infection, malignancy, chronic renal failure, or other disorders of the urinary tract.

Past Medical History. Ask about previous medical and surgical illnesses. Renal disorders are associated with a variety of metabolic, neurologic, GI, hematologic, dermatologic, skeletal, and respiratory disorders (discussed under Review of Systems).

Family History. The family history may reveal information related to structural anomalies of the urinary tract in other family members. An example is polycystic kidneys.

Psychosocial History and Lifestyle History. Assess factors related to the patient's lifestyle that may have a bearing on disorders of the urinary system. For instance, cigarette smoking and occupational exposure to substances, such as certain dyes, rubber, paint, and organic chemicals, have been found to increase the risk of bladder cancer. Episodes

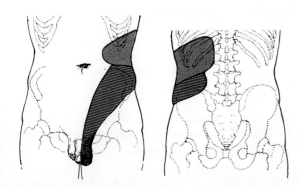

Figure 47–8. Referred pain from kidney (dotted areas) and ureter (shaded areas). (*From Tanagho and McAninch.*[79])

of calculi may be precipitated by dehydration that follows unusual physical exertion in hot weather. Another contributing factor may be the excessive intake of animal protein or vitamin D. The ingestion of certain medications, such as Pyridium, and foods, such as beets, may alter the composition and appearance of urine. Thus, obtain a relevant dietary and medication history, including the usual amount and type of daily fluid intake.

It is also important to determine if the presenting problem poses a threat to the individual's self-image or social functioning. For instance, incontinence may result in lowered self-esteem and interfere with social interactions. Incontinence may also affect sexual intercourse.

Review of Systems. Nurses need to be especially aware of (1) disorders in the urinary system that may affect other systems and (2) disorders in other systems that may affect urinary function. A few examples are listed.

Disorders in the Urinary System Affecting Other Systems. If the kidneys do not function correctly, changes in the *cardiovascular (CV) system* may occur. Fluid may be retained in the vascular system, resulting in increased blood pressure. The hypervolemia may also cause heart failure and pulmonary edema. Similarly, if the kidneys do not remove the waste products, such as blood urea nitrogen (BUN) and creatinine, from the blood normally, these substances will accumulate and cause *neurologic changes* such as decreased alertness, unconsciousness, and death. The *hematologic system* is affected in the patient with renal failure; anemia is related to decreased production of erythropoietin. Renal failure may cause bleeding in the *GI system* from the increased levels of gastrin.

Disorders in Other Systems Affecting the Urinary System. Recurrent or extended disorders of the *CV system,* such as cardiogenic or hypovolemic shock with associated hypotension, may result in decreased urine formation and result in renal failure. This condition can be fatal if effective intervention is not provided promptly. Changes in the blood vessels in the kidneys caused by diabetes mellitus, a disorder in the *endocrine system,* can lead to renal damage. The kidney is also a major site of damage from a disorder occurring in the *hematologic system* when a blood transfusion reaction occurs.

Contamination from the anal orifice of the *GI tract* may be the source of urethral and bladder infections in the female. Nephritis may be associated with a previous streptococcal infection of the throat. In the *male reproductive system,* enlargement of the prostate can contribute to urinary retention; the obstruction can eventually lead to damage of the entire urinary system if the obstruction is not relieved.

Physical Examination

General Inspection. During the interview, observe the patient for signs of renal insufficiency, including edema, particularly about the face and eyes, in the lower extremities, and, if the patient is bedfast, over the sacral area. Observe the skin turgor and status of hydration. Observe the skin color for pallor because patients with renal failure develop anemia.

Record vital signs, especially noting the temperature and blood pressure. An elevated temperature suggests a urinary tract infection, whereas an elevated blood pressure is a common manifestation of renal insufficiency.

A fullness in the flank may be observed when a renal tumor, cyst, or abscess is present, or when fluid has accumulated within the kidney pelvis (*hydronephrosis*). This bulging tends to be more prominent when the patient sits or leans forward.

A suprapubic bulge may be visible when the bladder is distended with 500 mL or more of urine. This observation is particularly important if the patient is unable to void or presents with a history of dribbling of urine.

Inspection of the patient's genitals may be necessary. If inspection is needed, observe the urinary meatus for edema, redness, and secretions.

Palpation. Because the *kidneys* are located deep within the upper abdominal cavity, palpation of the normal adult kidney may be impossible. The lower tip of the right kidney may be palpable because of the large area occupied by the liver. Place the patient in a supine position and stand at the patient's right side if you are right-handed. Place your left hand firmly on the patient's flank between the rib cage and the iliac crest, and elevate the patient's flank. Palpate the upper abdominal quadrants with the fingertips of your right hand, pressing just below the costal margin. Your fingertips should point laterally and slightly downward. Repeat the procedure with the other side. This examination is illustrated in Chap. 51 because palpation of the kidney is performed as part of the examination of the abdomen. The skilled examiner is sometimes able to "capture" the kidney between the two hands. If either kidney is palpated, note its size, general contour, and any tenderness encountered. It is not expected that the beginning examiner will be able to palpate the kidneys.

The *bladder* can be palpated only when it contains at least 150 mL of fluid. A round smooth bulge may then be felt in the suprapubic area when the patient is supine.

Percussion. Percussion techniques may be used to detect a distended bladder. Greatly distended bladders may be percussed as high as the umbilicus. Gentle fist percussion techniques over the costovertebral area may be used by the physician or an experienced nurse practitioner in assessing for possible renal tenderness. Percussion should *never* be used if the patient has polycystic kidneys or a renal transplant. Tenderness suggests the presence of infection.

Auscultation. Auscultate for bruits of the renal artery posteriorly at the area of the costovertebral angle and anteriorly over the upper abdominal quadrants.[6]

Summary. Table 47–4 lists key points of the physical examination.

TABLE 47–4

ASSESSMENT: KEY POINTS OF THE PHYSICAL EXAMINATION OF THE URINARY SYSTEM

Kidneys

By inspection assess for:
Presence of edema
Skin turgor
State of hydration
Pallor of the skin

By palpation
Attempt to palpate the kidneys (normally not palpable).

By auscultation
Assess for bruits over the renal arteries.

Bladder

By palpation
Assess for fullness and location of height of bladder.

By percussion
Percuss for bladder distention.
Assess for tenderness.

Urethral Meatus

By inspection
Assess for edema, redness, and the presence and characteristics of drainage.

Effects of Aging

A gradual reduction in renal mass (primarily cortical) and in the number of nephrons occurs after age 30. Many glomeruli become sclerotic and the afferent arterioles atrophy. The sclerotic nephrons are not replaced, but the remaining nephrons hypertrophy in an attempt to compensate for the functional loss. Between ages 25 and 85, the number of nephrons decreases about 30 to 40%. The net weight of the kidney decreases about 30% from maturity to old age.[27,34]

It is important to note that, although the creatinine clearance may be reduced by as much as 50%, the serum creatinine may be normal. This is because reduced muscle mass in the elderly results in less creatinine production. Therefore, it must not be assumed that if the serum creatinine of an elderly person is normal, the renal function is the same as that of a younger person with the same serum creatinine.

As a result of this decrease in renal function, the elderly may require altered doses of medications that are excreted primarily by the kidneys. They are also more susceptible to nephrotoxicity. Therefore, it is important to closely monitor the responses of an elderly patient to medications. The elderly are also at increased risk for renal damage secondary to uncontrolled hypertension, hypotension, obstruction, and urinary tract infection.

The older person will usually have some loss of bladder muscle tone: 14 to 40% have problems with urinary incontinence.[7] For undetermined reasons, there is a high incidence of frequency of urination and urgency incontinence in the elderly. Cerebral arteriosclerosis or other central nervous system pathology that results in an upper motor neuron type of neurogenic bladder may be a logical explanation. Detrusor contraction at socially inconvenient times and the inability to prevent urination through contraction of pelvic muscles and external sphincters may result in incontinence.

Immobility or decreased mobility is a problem of the elderly that leads to decreased muscle strength and loss of bladder muscle tone. The inefficiency of the detrusor muscle may lead to incomplete emptying of the bladder, and the presence of a cystocele in women promotes bacteriuria. This may explain the increased incidence of urinary tract infection in aging men and women. An enlarged prostate gland in the male may obstruct urine flow, causing urinary retention.

DIAGNOSTIC STUDIES

Diagnosis of disorders within the urinary system may involve a wide range of diagnostic studies. The studies discussed in this section include examination of the urine, tests of renal function, imaging techniques that outline the urinary tract or its vasculature, endoscopic studies of the urinary tract, and a biopsy of renal tissue. Although the diagnostic studies are requested by physicians, most studies require nursing interventions in preparing the patients and monitoring them for complications following the studies. The findings from diagnostic studies are used in planning the nursing management.

Nursing Management: Collection of Urine Specimens

Nurses are responsible for the collection of urine specimens, which may be accomplished by various means as described next.

First Voided Morning Specimen. To be useful, it is important that the urine specimen accurately reflect the characteristics of the urine in the bladder. The first voided morning urine is generally considered the ideal urine specimen because it is more concentrated and has a lower pH, permitting maximum observation of formed elements. A regularly voided specimen, after bathing the genitals to reduce surface contaminants, is satisfactory for most routine urinalyses. A midstream voided or a catheterized specimen is indicated if a bacteria count or culture is needed.[73]

Midstream Voided Urine Specimen. The procedure for collecting a midstream voided (also known as a *clean catch* or *clean voided*) urine sample is described in Table 47–5.

TABLE 47–5

PROCEDURES: COLLECTION OF URINE SPECIMENS: MIDSTREAM, FROM AN INDWELLING CATHETER, 24-HOUR SPECIMEN, AND RESIDUAL URINE

Note: Prior to preparation of the patient, collection of specimens, or handling of specimen containers, wash your hands and don non-sterile gloves.

Collection of Midstream Urine Specimen

1. *Female:* Keep the labia retracted throughout the procedure. *Male:* If not circumcised, keep the foreskin retracted throughout the procedure.

2. Cleanse the perineal area or glans penis gently with the cleansing solution provided by the individual institution (usually a dilute hexachlorine solution).

3. Rinse the area with water, so that the cleansing agent does not contaminate the specimen and alter results.

4. Before giving the collection container to the patient, label it with the patient's name and other identifying information. (It may be labeled after the specimen is collected.)

5. Instruct the patient to:
   a. Begin by voiding a small amount to wash out the distal urethra.
   b. Stop the stream briefly to position the collection container; if unable to stop, place the container in the stream.
   c. Continue voiding into the container until an adequate sample has been obtained (at least 10 mL if possible).
   d. Remove the container and complete the voiding into the urinal or toilet.

6. Cover the container securely as soon as the sample has been collected, and have it delivered to the laboratory promptly after collection.

Collection of Urine Specimen From an Indwelling Catheter

1. Explain the procedure to the patient.

2. If there is no urine in the catheter, kink the tubing about 3 in. below the catheter connection site and secure with a rubber band, thus allowing urine to collect. *This usually takes only a few minutes. Do not forget to release the tubing as soon as the specimen has been obtained.*

3. Clean the entry port carefully with an antiseptic swab.

4. Select a syringe of appropriate size (3 mL for a glucose/acetone test or a culture and sensitivity, 10 mL for routine urinalysis). Attach a small-gauge needle (21 to 25 gauge) to enhance self-sealing of the port site (Fig. 47–9).

5. Insert the needle into the catheter port at an angle to facilitate self-sealing. Slant the needle toward the drainage tubing to avoid accidentally puncturing the tubing to the retention balloon, thus deflating the balloon.

6. Aspirate the amount of urine needed; then carefully remove the needle.

7. *Release the tubing to allow unobstructed flow of urine to the drainage bag.*

8. Transfer the sample to the collection container that is labeled completely, and send to the laboratory immediately unless it has been collected for a test, such as acetone, which is usually performed on the unit.

Collection of 24-Hour Urine Specimen

Starting the Collection

1. Acquire the proper container and instructions for maintaining the container. In most institutions the laboratory supplies specially prepared and labeled gallon-size containers for 24-hour urine collections. Urine breaks down rapidly on standing, so these bottles usually contain a small, premeasured amount of preservative to retard the breakdown process. Depending on the purpose of the test, the 24-hour collection container may need to remain cool throughout the collection period. (Refer to the procedure of the agency for keeping the sample cool.)

2. Instruct the patient about the procedure.

3. The 24-hour urine collection period *begins with the bladder completely empty.* Instruct the patient to void; then discard the specimen unless it is being saved for another purpose. This specimen should *not* be poured into the collection container.

4. Record the exact time the bladder is emptied.

5. Instruct the patient to save each urine specimen.

6. *If a catheter is in place,* remove the drainage bag and connect the catheter to the specially prepared and labeled 24-hour collection bottle. Measure the amount of urine in the previous drainage bag and record the amount on the output record.

7. Post a notice prominently on the patient's bathroom door and other appropriate places so that urine will not be discarded accidentally.

Maintaining the Collection (If a Patient Does Not Have an Indwelling Catheter)

8. Place a special collection device over the rim of the commode; then lower the toilet seat. Remind the patient to use the collection container for each voiding. Stress that the loss of even a small amount of urine may alter the test findings.

9. Instruct the patient to notify the nursing personnel promptly after each voiding so that each specimen can be added to the 24-hour collection container soon after voiding.

Ending the Collection

10. End the collection *precisely* 24 hours after the patient's bladder was first emptied. For example, to start the collection, have the patient void initially at 10:00 AM and *discard* this sample; to end the collection have the patient void 24 hours later (10:00 AM on the following day) and *add* this last urine to the sample.

    As a safeguard, the patient may be alerted as to the closure time approximately an hour before the collection is to end and reminded to wait until the exact closure time before voiding.

11. *Add* the final specimen to the collection bottle, and record the exact closure time on the bottle and on the patient's chart.

12. Have the 24-hour collection transported to the laboratory.

Collection of Residual Urine

1. Explain to the patient that the physician wants to determine how much urine is remaining in the bladder after the patient voids. Inform the patient that, immediately after voiding, he or she will be catheterized with an indwelling catheter. If the amount of residual urine is more than the amount stated by the physician, which is often 100 mL, the indwelling catheter will remain in place. If it is less than the stated amount, the catheter will be removed.

2. Collect the equipment for placement of an indwelling catheter.

3. Advise the patient to inform you of the need to void.

4. Immediately after voiding, catheterize the patient.

5. Note the amount of urine obtained by catheterization. If it is the stated amount or more, inflate the balloon on the indwelling catheter and complete the procedure by connecting the catheter to the drainage bag and taping the catheter properly. If it is less than the stated amount, remove the catheter.

6. Record the amount of urine obtained in the patient's chart and whether the catheter was left in the bladder or removed.

Most adults can be instructed to perform this procedure satisfactorily with minimal assistance. A catheterized sample may be obtained if the patient is unable to urinate.

Collecting a Urine Specimen From an Indwelling Catheter.

When a patient has an indwelling catheter in place, the urine should be collected without disturbing the closed drainage system. Even briefly disconnecting the closed system greatly increases the risk of entry by infective organisms and the potential for a urinary tract infection. The sample should not be taken from the drainage bag, as the urine in the bag has remained for a time at room temperature, allowing bacteria to multiply and urine constituents to break down. Instead, the urine sample should be collected through the aspiration site (entry port) on the catheter (Fig. 47–9 and Table 47–5).

Collecting a 24-Hour Urine Specimen.

Whereas most urinalyses are performed on single voided specimens, it is sometimes necessary to examine a complete 24-hour urine sample. When needed, it is mandatory that the specimen include all of the urine the patient has voided during the designated 24-hour period (Table 47–5). If the patient does not have a urinary catheter in place, it is imperative that the patient's cooperation be obtained and that he or she fully understand the schedule. The nursing personnel providing care for the patient during this time must also understand the procedure.

Collecting Residual Urine.

Residual urine refers to urine remaining in the bladder immediately after voiding. It may remain in the bladder when there are disorders in the correct function of the bladder and urethra. Residual urine is usually not present with urethral stricture, although the urinary stream may be markedly impaired.[67] The method of collecting residual urine is described in Table 47–5.

Examination of the Urine

Examination of a urine specimen (urinalysis) is the most important tool in the diagnosis of urinary disorders. Although the specific diagnosis cannot always be determined through urinalysis, it is a preliminary step to guide the selection of further diagnostic efforts. Urinalysis is a relatively inexpensive diagnostic test that does not usually require an invasive procedure for sample collection.

Urinalysis. A urinalysis (also called UA or routine UA) refers to the gross and microscopic examination of a urine sample to determine the urinary pH and specific gravity and to identify the presence of abnormal substances.

Gross Examination. Normal urine varies in *color* from straw-colored to dark amber, depending on the mixture of pigments present and the dilution (ingestion of a large volume of fluids usually causes dilution). Freshly voided urine is usually clear, but may be cloudy in the absence of apparent pathology. Red or red-brown urine suggests the presence of blood (hematuria), whereas yellow-brown or green-brown urine often contains bile pigments. Numerous metabolic products, pigments, drugs (Pyridium, azulfidine, cascara), and foods (vegetables such as beets and food high in riboflavin) may also influence urine color.[73]

Fresh urine usually has an aromatic *odor*, but changes to the odor of ammonia if left standing. A sweet or fruity smell may be associated with acetone and acetoacetic acid formed during fasting, diabetes mellitus, and dehydration states. Heavily infected urine may have a particularly offensive odor.

Microscopic Examination. Microscopic examination provides a quick screening test for the presence of erythrocytes (red blood cells [RBCs]), leukocytes (white blood cells [WBCs]), bacteria, and other substances, therefore facilitat-

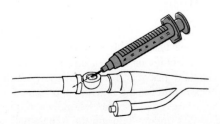

Figure 47–9. Obtaining urine specimen from aspiration port using sterile technique. (*From Norton and Miller.*[54])

ing earlier treatment. It also provides ongoing assessment of the effectiveness of therapy.

Reference values are as follows:

Bacteria	Less than 1 or 2 per high-powered field (hpf)
RBCs	Less than 2 or 3 per hpf
WBCs	Less than 4 or 5 per hpf
Crystals	A few may be present; usually have little clinical significance
Casts	Few hyaline casts (mixture of mucus and globulin congealed in the tubules); all others abnormal

The presence of more than two or three RBCs in the urine suggests that there is bleeding in the kidneys, in the lower urinary tract (ureters, bladder, urethra), or extra-renally (contamination with menstrual flow). The presence of RBCs and RBC casts together indicates infection or trauma within the kidney itself, whereas hematuria in the absence of RBC casts and proteinuria suggests bleeding of the lower urinary tract.

The number of WBCs increases markedly with all renal and urinary tract infections. A culture and sensitivity (C&S) test is usually indicated when a significant number of WBCs are found in the urine. Because of their short urethras, women are more likely than men to have urinary WBCs as a result of contamination of the external urinary meatus, and they also develop more urinary tract infections.

A few crystals do not signify disease. *Casts* are formed elements in the urine. Because casts are produced within the tubules, their presence (except for a few hyaline casts) always suggests a kidney disorder. Urinary casts have also been found in association with fever, exercise, and congestive heart failure. Granular casts usually represent disintegrated WBCs, epithelial cells, or protein and indicate a renal tubular disorder.[73,79]

Urinary pH. The urinary pH determines the acidity or alkalinity of the urine. The reference value is 4.5 to 8.0. A neutral pH is 7; values lower than 7 indicate acidity, whereas values higher than 7 indicate alkalinity. The procedure is performed by dipping a pH-sensitive paper strip into a urine sample. These commercially prepared dipsticks are available to assist persons monitoring the pH of their urine in an effort to discourage the development of urinary tract infections and prevent the formation of uric acid stones.

The urine pH reflects the plasma pH, so strongly acidic urine (4.5) suggests metabolic acidosis or diabetic acidosis. The recent ingestion of high-protein foods may cause a transient increase in urinary pH. Some medications (ammonium chloride and mandelic acid) may also produce a low urine pH. Alkaline urine (7.5) suggests the presence of urea-splitting bacteria such as *Proteus mirabilis,* metabolic alkalosis as seen with severe vomiting, or the recent ingestion of alkalinizing medications, such as soda bicarbonate, or low-protein foods, such as vegetables.[73]

Specific Gravity. Specific gravity (*sp gr*) is a comparison of the density of urine with the density of water (1.000). The

higher the number, the more concentrated the urine—the greater the number of dissolved solutes present. The reference value is a specific gravity from 1.001 to 1.030.

A low value, such as 1.005, with dilute urine suggests that (1) there has been a large intake of water or (2) the kidneys are unable to concentrate the urine, as occurs in diabetes insipidus and distal renal tubular disease.

An elevated value, such as 1.028, with concentrated urine occurs (1) when the volume is depleted as during dehydration, because the kidneys conserve fluid; (2) with conditions in which there are increased solutes in the urine, such as diabetes mellitus with increased glucose in the urine; and (3) with the contrast medium used for some x-ray studies.

Protein. Protein in the urine is most often checked by the dipstick method. Other laboratory procedures are available if a more specific protein analysis is necessary. The reference value for protein in the urine is none normally. *Proteinuria* refers to protein in the urine.

Detection of protein in the urine is a serious finding and is an indication that more specific diagnostic studies need to be initiated. Persistent proteinuria is associated with renal disorders. Albumin is the protein usually lost, but other types of protein are seen in myelomas. In the nephrotic syndrome, as much as 3,500 to 20,000 mg of protein may be lost through the urine daily.

Glucose. Glycosuria or glucosuria refers to the presence of glucose in the urine. The reference value for glucose in the urine is none. The usual renal threshold for glucose is approximately 160 to 200 mg/dL. This means that no glucose appears in the urine until the blood sugar rises above that level. Diabetes mellitus may cause an increased blood sugar as well as alter the renal threshold for glucose. Patients on hyperalimentation may have glycosuria if the solution infuses at a faster rate than insulin can be produced.

Acetone (Ketone Bodies). Urine acetone is measured using a dipstick or tablets. The reference value for acetone in the urine (ketonuria) is none. Excess acetone (also called *ketone*) is formed when carbohydrate metabolism is altered so that fat becomes the main body fuel. Acetone is usually measured at the same time that routine glucose tests are done to determine if body fat or protein is being oxidized to provide energy. Ketonuria is most often associated with diabetes, and may also be associated with fever, starvation, low food intake, diarrhea, prolonged vomiting, or anesthesia.[25]

Nursing Management: Urinalysis. If a sample of urine is noted to have an unusual color or odor, a check should be done to see if the patient has received medications or foods that could be responsible for the unusual appearance. If so, this information is recorded on the laboratory request. If the urine sample was obtained during the female patient's menstrual flow, this should be recorded because there is an increased chance that the sample could be contaminated with blood.

If for some reason the urine cannot be examined immediately, it should be refrigerated. If urine is allowed to stand at room temperature for more than 30 minutes, sediment in the urine is altered, RBCs break down, and casts disintegrate as the urine becomes alkaline. Bacteria may enter the container and multiply, leading to an incorrect diagnosis of infection.

If the individual is taking a drug, such as a sulfa preparation, that is known to cause crystals in the urine, the nurse should note and confer with the physician about a report of crystal formation. Unless contraindicated, the patient should be encouraged to increase fluid intake to 2.5 to 3 L daily while receiving medication.

Although glycosuria is a classic symptom of diabetes mellitus, it may also occur as an isolated event unrelated to diabetes, such as the recent ingestion of a large amount of glucose or exposure to a stressor (trauma). Thus, it is important that health professionals not immediately conclude that the patient with glycosuria is diabetic, but that the patient be encouraged to have follow-up visits.

If glycosuria is caused by hyperalimentation fluids infusing too rapidly, the nurse confers with the physician about decreasing the rate. The increased glucose acts as an osmotic diuretic, causing extra water to be excreted as urine. If it is not realistic to decrease the flow rate, regular insulin is sometimes infused in a separate intravenous solution or is administered on a sliding-scale basis to control the glycosuria.

Unless contraindicated, additional fluids are offered frequently to any patient with glycosuria from any cause to prevent dehydration. Fluid intake is also encouraged following an x-ray procedure in which contrast medium was used.

Urine Osmolality. Urine osmolality is a determination of the total number of particles in the urine without regard to the size or weight of the particles. Osmolality is based on the freezing point of a solution; thus, the value is recorded in "osmoles," a standard of measurement based on the freezing point of a solution.

Because urine osmolality does not vary with dietary intake and changes in urine content, it is a more accurate measure of urine concentration than is specific gravity. This test is used when specific gravity or other renal tests suggest a problem related to the ability of the kidney to concentrate urine. A high osmolality suggests dehydration. A comparison of urine and serum osmolality may also be helpful in establishing diagnoses. The reference values and clinical implications of changes in serum and urine osmolality are summarized in Table 47–6.

Diagnostic Studies of Renal Function Performed on Serum

Unless stated otherwise, a 1-mL sample of blood or serum for each test is chemically analyzed.

Blood Urea Nitrogen (BUN). BUN is a measure of the amount of urea nitrogen in the blood. The reference value is 5 to 20 mg/dL. Urea is cleared from the bloodstream by the kidneys. Because of the strong association between increased urea levels in the blood and the clinical findings associated with renal disorders, BUN is a commonly used renal function test.

BUN values vary widely according to the dietary intake of protein, but values *elevated* to more than 20 mg/dL suggest renal insufficiency or excessive breakdown of body protein as may occur with sepsis, fever, dehydration, shock, congestive heart failure, or GI bleeding. Specific disorders of the kidney associated with an elevated BUN include glomerulonephritis, pyogenic infections, and trauma. In case of renal parenchymal disease, an increased BUN does not occur until the function of approximately two thirds of

TABLE 47–6

CLINICAL IMPLICATIONS OF CHANGES IN OSMOLALITY

Serum Osmolality (282–295 mOsm)	Urine Osmolality (500–800 mOsm)	Clinical Significance
Normal or increased	Increased	Fluid volume deficit
Decreased	Decreased	Fluid volume excess
Normal	Decreased	1. Increased fluid intake or 2. Diuretic use
Increased or normal	Decreased (with no increase in fluid intake)	1. Kidneys unable to concentrate urine 2. Lack of ADH (diabetes insipidus)
Decreased	Increased	Syndrome of inappropriate secretion of ADH (SIADH) can be caused by stress, trauma, drugs, or malignancies

(Source: *Corbett.*[17])

the nephrons has been lost. A *decreased* BUN may be associated with overhydration, malnutrition, and severe liver disease. BUN levels are also used to monitor renal function in persons who are receiving drugs that are known to be toxic to the kidneys, such as aminoglycosides.

Creatinine. Creatinine is a waste product in the blood, originating from creatine as it participates in the physiology of skeletal muscle contraction. Both the creatine level in the body and therefore the creatinine level in the blood remain constant and are not affected by dietary intake, status of hydration, or other factors that alter the BUN level. The reference value is 0.5 to 1.5 mg/dL. Individuals with larger muscle mass may have slightly higher creatinine levels.[73]

An *elevated* serum creatinine occurs in all kidney disease in which 50% of the nephrons are destroyed. Damage to a large number of nephrons is the primary pathologic condition that causes a significant increase in serum creatinine, so it is a much more specific test for renal dysfunction than BUN.[79] Persons with unusually large muscle mass or those with acromegaly may have slightly elevated serum creatinine levels. Serum creatinine levels are frequently used to monitor the success of drug therapy, dialysis, and renal transplants, and also to detect possible renal damage when nephrotoxic drugs, such as the aminoglycoside antibiotics, are being administered.

A *decreased* serum creatinine level suggests atrophy of muscle tissue. A serum creatine test would be indicated as a more definitive test for problems involving skeletal muscles.

BUN/Creatinine Ratio. A comparison of BUN with the serum creatinine level (BUN/creatinine ratio) is often more helpful in assessing renal dysfunction than BUN alone because the creatinine level is altered only by renal disorders. The reference value is 10:1 to 15:1. An increased ratio suggests dehydration or protein breakdown. A decreased ratio may reflect a low intake of protein, overhydration, or severe liver disease.

Nursing Management. Because an elevated *BUN* may reflect significant renal disorders or damage, the nurse may expect prescribed measures to lessen the work of the kidney (low-protein diet, fluid management, and possibly dialysis) and to correct disorders as much as possible.[36] The report of the BUN level should be checked before administering a drug known to be potentially toxic to the kidneys. Occasionally a drug will be prescribed that is known to be nephrotoxic and is administered even with increased BUN levels, because the physician thinks the potential benefit outweighs the risk. If the increased BUN is a new finding, the nurse confers with the physician before administering the drug.

Because *creatinine* is not elevated until half of the nephrons are nonfunctioning, patients with elevated creatinine are likely to have severe renal impairment. The nursing management may need to be adjusted quickly to address the many crucial nursing problems associated with renal insufficiency or failure. There is also a serum creatine test that is

used to evaluate degenerative disorders of muscles, and so a check is done that the correct test is requested on the laboratory slip.

Creatinine Clearance. Creatinine clearance is a test that compares the serum creatinine level with the amount of creatinine excreted in a volume of urine during a specified period. The reference value is 72 to 140 mL/min.

In this procedure, a 24-hour urine collection must be obtained as outlined in Table 47–5. Abbreviated procedures with 2-hour or 12-hour collections may also be used. A blood sample is drawn near the midpoint of the collection period. Creatinine values are determined for the serum and urine and the exact volume is recorded for the 24-hour urine collection. The rate of creatinine clearance is then determined by placing the values in the following formula:

$$\frac{\text{urine creatinine} \times \text{urine volume}}{\text{serum creatinine}} = \text{creatinine clearance rate}$$

The rate is expressed in milliliters per minute, with a mathematical correction for body size. Because the creatinine clearance value reflects the glomerular filtration rate and is relatively easy to obtain, it is the *most accurate measure of renal function* in common use.

This test is based on the premise that creatinine is excreted by glomerular filtration and is *not* reabsorbed or secreted by the tubule cells. The major advantage of the creatinine clearance test is that it detects renal disorders in earlier stages than is possible with serum creatinine values alone. Creatinine clearance tests may also be used to evaluate the progression of renal disease. A decreased creatinine clearance rate indicates decreased glomerular function.

Nursing Management. The most crucial aspect is to elicit the patient's cooperation in the 24-hour urine collection. If some of the urine is lost, the result may be a false low reading. The implications for nursing management for the patient with a decreased creatinine clearance rate depend on the severity of the renal disorder and related long-term plans.

Uric Acid. Uric acid is a measure of the end-product of purine metabolism. The reference value is 2 to 7 mg/dL. Purines, which are located in all cells, are obtained from dietary sources and from the breakdown of body proteins. Uric acid is excreted as a waste product. The level considered pathologic is controversial because there have been wide "normal" ranges, and there are daily and seasonal variations in levels.

Elevated levels occur consistently in patients with gout. Increased values also occur in patients with renal impairment; but the levels do not correlate with the severity of the renal disease and so are not used to test renal function. Elevations may occur with abnormal cell destruction, such as in neoplasms; or with use of chemotherapy or radiation therapy. An elevation may be present in patients with chronic malnutrition or prolonged fasting.[36] An elevation also occurs in hemolytic anemia.

Although the association is unclear, an elevation of uric acid with hyperlipidemia and coronary artery disease has sometimes been observed. Some drugs, such as the thiazides and other diuretics, can impair uric acid clearance by the kidneys and cause an elevation. Decreased levels are not considered clinically important; they usually represent increased plasma volume.

Serum Osmolality. The major substances that determine the osmolality of extracellular fluid are (1) sodium and its accompanying anions, (2) glucose, and (3) urea. Various formulas are used to calculate osmolality. By using the following formula, the serum osmolality can be approximately measured.[73]

Serum osmolality (mOsm/L)

$$= 2Na + \frac{glucose\ (mg/dL)}{18} + \frac{BUN\ (mg/dL)}{2.8}$$

Sodium is multiplied by 2 to account for its accompanying anions (such as chloride or bicarbonate). Serum osmolality is measured in milliosmoles per liter (mOsm/L). To convert the mg/dL of glucose and BUN to mOsm/L, glucose is divided by its molecular weight of 18 and urea nitrogen is divided by its molecular weight of 2.8.

The reference value for serum osmolality is 280 to 300 mOs/L.[36] Coma may occur at elevations greater than 325 mOm/L.[29]

Serum osmolality is used to determine fluid balance. It can be used in conjunction with urine osmolality to determine renal function. Table 47–6 lists clinical implications of changes in osmolality. *Nursing management* is related to the underlying disorder(s) causing the changes in osmolality.

Imaging Techniques to Outline the Urinary Tract or Its Vasculature

Many highly complex techniques are available to produce images of parts of the urinary system or their vasculature. Because many of these techniques are also used to assess other body systems, they are described in Chap. 4.

Plain Abdominal X-Ray. The plain abdominal x-ray is also called a *flat plate* or *survey film of the abdomen*. It is also called a *KUB* (acronym for the kidneys, ureters, and bladder), although the ureters are not visible unless they contain calculi. The KUB, the initial step in imaging studies, may show the kidneys and a distended bladder. *Uses* include indicating the presence of calculi or ruling out general abdominal disorders, such as intestinal obstruction or gas. It is often combined with more definitive x-ray examinations using radiopaque material to facilitate structural and functional assessment of the urinary tract.

In the *procedure,* an x-ray is made of the abdomen. Related *nursing management* usually includes administering a prescribed laxative or enema to empty the bowel to allow better visualization. This procedure is not invasive and requires no contrast medium, and so special follow-up nursing care is not required related to the x-ray. The care for the patient will depend on the problem causing the need for this study.

Excretory Urogram. An excretory urogram (formerly called an *intravenous pyelogram* or *IVP*) is a series of x-rays performed after the intravenous injection of radiopaque dye allows visualization of the renal parenchyma, filling of renal pelves, and outline of the ureters and bladder. Its *uses* are to provide an accurate assessment of the excretory function of the kidneys and the structural integrity of the kidneys, ureters, and bladder. It is particularly useful in the diagnosis of a variety of urinary tract lesions.

For the *procedure,* a preliminary abdominal x-ray (KUB) is taken, and then the patient receives a rapid intravenous injection of a radiopaque dye that will be excreted by the kidneys. X-rays are taken at postinjection intervals, possibly at 1, 5, and 10 minutes. Another film is made at 20 minutes to visualize the bladder. A postvoiding film is made if the patient is suspected of having residual urine.

Unfortunately, a number of potential *complications* are associated with this procedure. Occasionally a patient may have a serious allergic (anaphylactic) reaction to the contrast medium.

The radiology staff is alert to signs of allergic reactions, particularly during the first 5 minutes after the injection. A physician should be present during the procedure, and appropriate medications (such as adrenalin), oxygen, and resuscitation equipment should be available for immediate use in the event of an allergic reaction.

This procedure may be done on an outpatient basis. If the patient is hospitalized, related *nursing management* is to instruct the patient about nursing aspects of the procedure. Because any accumulation of feces or flatus in the intestines may obstruct the view of the kidneys in the x-rays, the bowel is usually cleansed by administering a prescribed cathartic, cleansing enema, or both on the evening before the procedure. Slight dehydration favors a greater concentration of dye in the kidney, and so the patient should receive nothing by mouth after midnight. To allow adequate visualization, an excretory urogram should be scheduled before any procedure involving barium swallows or enemas.

It is especially important to inform the patient that a brief, transient warm flushing feeling of the face and a salty taste may be noticed as the dye is injected. Prior to the procedure, the patient is questioned about previous allergic reactions to shellfish, contrast media, or other iodine-containing preparations. If a history of such an allergy is revealed, notify the physician. The female patient is questioned about being pregnant.

Once the procedure has been completed, the patient continues to be observed for allergies. If allergic symptoms (Table 4–4) are present, the physician is notified immediately. If allowed, increased fluid intake is encouraged to rid the kidneys of the contrast medium and to prevent hypotension related to hypovolemia. The vital signs and urine output are monitored closely after the procedure.

Cystography and Urethrography. A cystography and urethrography are a series of x-rays of the bladder and urethra after instillation of radiopaque fluid into the bladder through a urethral catheter. Their *uses* are to provide information about the structure and function of the lower urinary tract. Retrograde and delayed cystograms specifically outline a diverticulum (a pouchlike protrusion) or a fistula (an abnormal tubelike passage) between the bladder and vagina. The voiding cystourethrogram is used to detect urethral reflux (backward flow of urine into the bladder) or urethral strictures. Urethrograms outline the shape and size of the urethra, thus detecting stenosis of the urethra, enlargement of the prostate, diverticula, fistulas, and other structural abnormalities of the urethra.

During the *procedure,* after a preliminary KUB is obtained, a catheter is inserted to drain the urine. Approximately 200 to 300 mL of a solution containing a radiopaque dye is instilled into the bladder. The catheter is clamped; then a series of x-rays (retrograde cystograms) are taken with the patient in supine, lateral, and sitting positions. The dye is drained and another x-ray (delayed cystogram) is taken.

For a cystourethrogram, radiopaque fluid is instilled into the bladder and the urethra; then x-rays are taken. To obtain a voiding cystourethrogram, the patient is instructed to void, and x-rays are made during the micturition process. A retrograde urethrogram consists of an x-ray taken while a radiopaque lubricant is being instilled into the urethra.[25]

Visualization of the Urinary Tract

Cystoscopy and Urethroscopy. Cystoscopy and unrethroscopy constitute a direct method of visualizing the internal portions of the urinary structures through a lighted instrument (cystoscope) inserted through the urethra. The tests are useful in determining the presence of inflammation, tumors, stones, or structural irregularities in the lining of the urethra or bladder. Enlargement in adjacent structures, such as the prostate, may also be detected.

For the *procedure,* the patient is placed in a lithotomy position; then the cystoscope is inserted through the urethra, usually under local anesthesia. A sedative may be given before the procedure begins. If local anesthesia is used, the patient should be informed that a strong urge to void may be felt during this procedure.

The bladder is completely inspected with special attention to the presence of trabeculation, cellules (Fig. 49–2), or diverticula that may contain stagnant urine. The neck of the bladder is examined for evidence of bar formation (bars around the bladder neck), intrusion of the prostate into the bladder, and an estimate of the prostate size. To determine if the prostate is occluding the bladder, the bladder is filled with sterile water and the cystoscope is gradually withdrawn while the bladder neck opening is observed.

During this procedure a *retrograde pyelogram* may also be performed in which catheters are passed through the ureters. Urine samples may be collected and dye is injected into the renal pelves to outline the renal collecting system and examine it for filling defects.

A significant number of men undergoing cystoscopy have been reported to experience the *complication* of arrhythmias, perhaps resulting from stimulation of the sympathetic and parasympathetic nerves within the urinary tract. Cystoscopy is delayed when an acute urinary tract infection is present to prevent its exacerbation. Likewise, it is not used in patients with severe prostatic obstruction, as the trauma it produces may worsen the condition.

Cystoscopy is considered an uncomfortable procedure and requires adequate support and instruction of the patient. If the patient is to have general anesthesia, *nursing management* includes instruction that nothing be taken by mouth after midnight prior to the procedure, and intravenous fluids may be started to ensure adequate urine flow for specimens.

Pink-tinted urine is expected after the procedure, and the patient is assessed for excessive hematuria, bladder spasms, lower back discomfort, burning and frequency on urination, elevated temperature, and a feeling of bladder fullness. The prescribed mild analgesics, Sitz baths, and increased fluid intake that help to relieve these symptoms are provided. Urine output and vital signs are monitored carefully during the postprocedure period.

Urodynamic Studies

Urodynamic studies evaluate bladder function and voiding problems by measuring pressure, urinary flow, and striated muscle activity. The four basic components of urodynamics are (1) uroflowmetry, (2) cystometrogram, (3) electromyography, and (4) urethral pressure profile. These studies are used in various combinations to provide important information about the micturition process and common abnormalities. Urodynamic study is an area of testing still being developed.[79]

Uroflowmetry. Uroflowmetry or voiding flow rate measurement (Fig. 47–10) uses a specially equipped commode chair that is provided with a button the patient pushes to start the machine when urination begins, eliminating the need to be observed. As the patient voids, characteristics of the voided stream are recorded, along with calculations related to peak and average flow rates (Fig. 47–10). For a valid recording the adult must void 200 to 400 mL. This test provides information related to a disorder caused by a neurogenic bladder or benign prostatic hypertrophy. Reference values are peak flow greater than 15 mL/sec and average flow rate greater than 12 mL/sec. The normal flow pattern (Fig. 47–10A) is a bell-shaped curve without interruptions or sharp peaks, sustained for over 20 seconds.

Cystometrogram. A cystometrogram (CMG) is a measure of bladder pressure during both bladder filling and voiding. The bladder is filled with either carbon dioxide or sterile water and a continuous recording is made of the pressure during the filling and subsequent voiding. The patient is asked to note two sensations: the first sensation of filling and the second sensation of fullness (urge to void). At the end of the procedure, the patient is asked to strain; the effects of abdominal pressure on the bladder pressure are as-

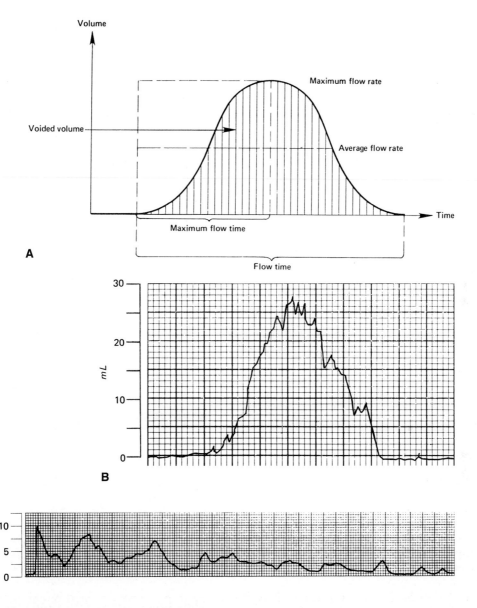

Figure 47–10. Uroflowmetry. **A.** Basic elements of maximum flow, average flow, total flow time, and total volume voided. **B.** Classic normal flow rate, with peak of about 30 mL/sec and average of about 20 mL/sec. **C.** Classic low flow rate of bladder outlet obstruction (benign prostatic hypertrophy), markedly prolonged flow time, and fluctuation resulting from attempt to improve flow by increasing intra-abdominal pressure. In **B** and **C** on the horizontal scale, one large square equals 5 seconds. (*From Tanagho and McAninch.*[79])

sessed. Most patients report a sensation of fullness between 100 and 300 mL and have the urge to void at approximately 400 to 500 mL. Information obtained from this test can be used to plan fluid intake and schedule effective times to stimulate voiding or intermittent catheterization. CMG is also advised in the work-up of women with urgency and stress incontinence. Determining the cause of incontinence can help to determine the treatment regimen.

Electromyography. Electromyography (EMG) is the study of electrical events that occur in striated muscles in the per-

ineal area, including the sphincters, during micturition. Electrodes record electrical activity in the muscles. In combination with other urodynamic testing, this test can assist in evaluating the neuromuscular coordinating activity of spinal and cerebellar reflex centers.

Urethral Pressure Profile. A urethral pressure profile (UPP) is used to evaluate the activity of smooth muscle surrounding the urethra. A small catheter is inserted through which water or carbon dioxide is infused. As the infusion continues, the catheter is slowly withdrawn using an automated puller mechanism; resistance exerted by the urethral wall is recorded on graph paper. The profile provides information concerning smooth muscle tone along the urethra. Low pressure readings suggest incontinence, whereas very high readings suggest excessive muscle tone that may be related to retention. Scars or strictures in the urethra produce high readings.

Nursing Management: Urodynamic Studies. Health professionals should be aware of and support studies of urodynamic testing so that they may inform patients appropriately. It is in this research area that potential solutions are being found for the troublesome urinary problems that hamper the lifestyles for many otherwise independent individuals and for individuals with neurologic problems.

Biopsy of Renal Tissue

In a biopsy of the kidney (also called a *renal mass puncture*), a sample of renal tissue is obtained for microscopic examination. *Uses* are (1) to aid in diagnosing diseases that alter the structure of the glomeruli, (2) to monitor the course of a chronic renal disease, and (3) to determine whether a mass is a tumor, clot, or stone.

For the *procedure*, postbiopsy bleeding is a serious concern, and so prebiopsy hematocrit and bleeding and clotting tests are always obtained. Under local anesthesia and with needle insertion usually monitored by fluoroscopy or scanning, a specially designed needle is inserted into the cortex of the kidney and a very small sample of tissue is obtained. The patient is asked to take a breath and hold it while the needle is being inserted to prevent unnecessary injury. A pressure dressing is applied immediately to prevent bleeding.

Nursing management prebiopsy includes withholding food and fluids before the procedure. The patient is often anxious; information presented by the physician about the procedure is reinforced by the nurse. Baseline vital signs are recorded.

Postbiopsy, the patient is instructed to lie still for 4 hours to prevent bleeding, and a sandbag may be placed on the biopsy site. Bed rest is enforced for at least 24 hours. Vital signs are monitored, the dressing is checked, the urine is monitored for hematuria, and fluid intake is encouraged regularly during the first 24 hours. The hematocrit is checked every 8 hours. The patient is instructed to avoid strenuous or jarring activities for several days and to immediately report flank pain, burning on urination, hematuria, dizziness, or weakness. Because infection can occur after a biopsy, temperature should be monitored carefully for a few days.

■ NURSING DIAGNOSES/COLLABORATIVE PROBLEMS AND PLANNING

Nursing diagnoses/collaborative problems that are frequently applicable when planning nursing care for patients with problems of the urinary system are listed below, along with examples of possible related etiologies. The examples

are not intended to be complete; other diagnoses may also apply, depending on each patient's actual situation. Based on these diagnoses, the nursing management is planned. Suggestions are listed in the plans in this unit on the urinary system.

- *Individual coping, ineffective* related to chronic illness, change in self-esteem or body image, lack of support
- *Fluid volume excess* related to renal failure, excess sodium intake, medication regimen
- *Grieving, anticipatory,* related to impending loss of life or decrease in independence
- *Incontinence* (*urge, stress, reflex, functional, or total*) related to incompetent bladder outlet, weakened pelvic muscles and structural supports, neurologic dysfunction, infectious process
- *Nutrition, more than body requirements, altered* related to actual or potential toxicity from elevated potassium or edema from excess sodium retention
- *Pain* related to renal calculi, surgery, or diagnostic procedures
- *Self-care deficit* (*toileting*) related to incontinence
- *Skin integrity, risk for impaired,* related to constant moisture caused by incontinence or irritation due to infection
- *Urinary elimination, altered patterns,* related to urinary tract infection, calculi, and decreased muscle tone/neurogenic control

■ INTERVENTION AND EVALUATION

Professional nurses provide care for patients that aids them in preserving the function of the urinary system. They also support patients with urinary problems when they feel anxious and out of control over one of the basic functions in life—elimination of urine. This section is divided into three subsections related to the nursing care for patients who have (1) problems related to renal insufficiency, (2) problems requiring urethral catheterization, and (3) urinary incontinence.

CARE OF PATIENTS WITH RENAL INSUFFICIENCY

Patients with abnormal renal function may develop multiple problems because of the complex functions of the kidneys. Nursing management related to these problems is described in Table 47–7. Corticosteroid and immunosuppressive therapy may be used as one type of treatment; potential problems and related nursing management are discussed in Table 47–8.

Evaluation/Desired Outcomes. The patient with abnormal renal function:

1. And fluid imbalance will maintain a satisfactory adjustment between intake and output
2. And electrolyte imbalances will select appropriate foods
3. And problems with maintaining a normal urinary output will comply with the prescribed dietary protein intake and will maintain fluid intake as prescribed
4. Will preserve renal function by learning about the disease, report for follow-up care when problems develop, take ap-

TABLE 47–7

NURSING MANAGEMENT PLAN: THE PATIENT WITH RENAL INSUFFICIENCY

Potential Nursing Diagnoses/Collaborative Problems
- *Fluid volume excess or deficit related to diminished renal blood flow*
- *Urinary elimination, altered, related to fluid and electrolyte imbalance*
- *Protection, altered, related to loss of plasma proteins that contain antibodies or to uremia*
- *Skin integrity, risk for impaired related to retention of waste products*

Goals/Desired Outcomes
- *The patient will (a) maintain adequate fluid and electrolyte balance, (b) maintain adequate urinary output and elimination, (c) preserve renal function, (d) avoid infections, and (e) maintain intact skin by appropriate treatment and self-care measures.*

Interventions	Rationale/Significance
A. Problems With Abnormal Fluid Balance	
Hypervolemia	
1. Weigh the patient daily or more often if indicated. Use the metric scale if possible.	1. An overnight weight gain usually reflects water retention; 1 kg (2.2 lb) = 1 L water. Therefore, weight can be converted to an estimation of the amount of fluid retained.
2. Monitor the blood pressure and pulse in lying, sitting, and standing positions (if possible). Wait approximately 5 minutes between each reading. Note the pulse, rhythm, and regularity.	2. A drop in blood pressure of more than 10 mm Hg from one position to the next is considered a significant *orthostatic* change. An increase in pulse of 20 to 30 beats per minute on position change is also significant and may precede a drop in blood pressure.
3. Monitor the respiratory status. Assess the respiratory rate, characteristics of the respirations, and breath sounds. Note the quantity and character of sputum.	3. Tachypnea may be associated with fluid volume excess. The presence of crackles and wheezes indicates pulmonary congestion. Fluid can also accumulate in the pleural cavity and cause pain on respiration and decreased breath sounds over the area. A pulmonary friction rub may also be present and is associated with renal failure.
4. Monitor the heart sounds. Note the rate, rhythm, and presence of an S_3, S_4, or pericardial friction rub.	4. The onset of an S_3 is associated with heart failure and is an important clinical finding. An S_4 is associated with hypertension. A pericardial friction rub may be associated with renal failure and may cause pain. Pericardial effusion may also occur and may be detected by an echocardiogram.
5. Assess the neck veins with the patient sitting at a 45-degree angle. Measure the vertical distance in centimeters between the level of venous pulsation and sternal angle (Chap. 19).	5. Intravascular fluid volume excess is associated with venous congestion and engorged neck veins. In fluid volume excess associated with decreased intravascular volume and increased interstitial fluid, the neck veins may be "flat," even in the supine position. In fluid volume deficit, the neck veins are also flat.
6. Note periorbital, pedal, pretibial, and sacral areas for edema. If ascitic fluid is also accumulating, measure the circumference of the abdomen.	6. Edema is usually first noted in dependent areas. In hypoproteinemic states, fluid may also accumulate in the abdomen and produce ascites.
7. Maintain accurate records of intake and output (I&O). Compare findings. • Administer prescribed IV medications in the smallest amount of fluid possible. • Distribute the oral intake throughout 24 hours. • Maintain the prescribed restriction. • Plan fluid intake schedule with the patient. • Avoid placing a water pitcher at the bedside. • Encourage good oral hygiene.	7. I&O records are important in evaluating the fluid status; however, weight is the *most accurate* indicator of volume status.
8. Administer prescribed diuretic.	8. A diuretic may be prescribed to assist in fluid elimination.
9. Monitor the serum and urinary sodium, serum osmolality, and hematocrit.	9. A patient with fluid retention may have a "dilution hyponatremia" and a drop in serum osmolality and hematocrit directly related to the excess fluid. Urinary electrolytes are important in the evaluation of tubular function.

(Continued)

TABLE 47–7   *(Continued)*

NURSING MANAGEMENT PLAN: THE PATIENT WITH RENAL INSUFFICIENCY

Interventions	Rationale/Significance
10. Consult with the physician about any changes that may indicate a deterioration of renal and/or cardiovascular function.	10. The following are reported promptly: • Weight gain greater than 5 lb in 24 hours • Orthostatic changes in blood pressure and pulse • Tachypnea • Development of wheezes and crackles or decreased breath sounds • Development of S_3, pericardial friction rub, or irregular pulse • Decrease in urine output
11. Provide psychologic support to the patient and family.	11. Fluid retention can precipitate anxiety and changes in body image.

Hypovolemia

1. Maintain accurate records of daily weights and of all forms of fluid intake and all forms of output. Compare the findings; notify the physician of significant variations. Consult with the physician if the *urine output is less than 30 mL hourly.*	1. These records are essential in determining fluid status. *Insensible loss* averages about 500 mL per day but may be considerably more. Insensible loss is that volume of fluid lost through the lungs and evaporation from the skin.
2. Monitor the blood pressure and pulse. Use the same procedure outlined under Hypervolemia.	2. Orthostatic changes increase as volume decreases (discussed under Hypervolemia). Hypotension is usually seen in volume depletion; however, in renin-dependent states, early volume depletion may be seen in conjunction with some degree of hypertension.
3. Monitor for signs of hypovolemia: dry skin, decreased skin turgor, dry mucous membranes, sunken eyeballs, flat neck veins. Provide good skin care and oral hygiene.	3. Fluid volume deficit affects intravascular, interstitial, and intracellular spaces.
4. Monitor laboratory studies, including hematocrit, sodium, potassium, BUN, creatinine, BUN:creatinine ratio, and urinary electrolytes. Consult with the physician about significant findings.	4. Because of volume depletion, the hematocrit and serum sodium may be elevated. Depending on the renal and metabolic status, serum potassium may be increased or decreased, and the BUN, creatinine, and ratio of the two may change.
5. Administer prescribed fluids, either orally or intravenously, or by both routes.	5. The best route to replace fluids is orally if nausea and vomiting are not present and the patient is able to drink. If fluids and electrolytes need to be replaced rapidly, the intravenous route is also used.
6. Provide psychologic support to the patient and family.	6. The patient and family are frequently anxious about the patient's current and future health status.

B. Problems With Maintaining Electrolyte Balance

Sodium

1. Monitor serum and urinary sodium levels. Consult with the physician about abnormal levels (reference values: serum Na$^+$, 135–145 mEq/L; urine Na$^+$, 100 mEq/L). Serum Na$^+$ levels less than 120 mEq require prompt treatment.	1. Hypernatremia and hyponatremia may be associated with renal abnormalities. Hyponatremia related to excess water is most common.
2. Monitor the weight and the intake and output closely. For hypernatremia related to volume deficit, encourage water intake and/or restrict salt intake. For hyponatremia related to water excess, limit the water intake; adhere to the physician's prescription for fluid intake carefully.	2. Serum sodium changes in response to free water load. It is *important* that hyponatremia be corrected very carefully and slowly.
3. Monitor for signs and symptoms of sodium abnormalities: *hypernatremia*—thirst, oliguria, confusion, lethargy, muscle weakness, twitching, convulsions, and coma; *hyponatremia*—malaise, nausea and vomiting, headache, confusion, lethargy, convulsions, and coma.	3. Sodium imbalances cause osmotic changes in serum and cells.

Interventions	Rationale/Significance

Potassium

1. Monitor serum potassium (K⁺) levels. Report any significant abnormal levels to the physician (reference values: serum K⁺, 3.6–5.5 mEq/L; urinary K⁺, 90 mEq/L).

2. Monitor the patient for symptoms of potassium imbalance: *hyperkalemia*—abdominal pain, vomiting, muscle weakness, flaccid paralysis, cardiac arrhythmias; *hypokalemia*—muscle weakness, cardiac arrhythmias, cardiac arrest.

3. Implement K⁺ replacement or restriction as prescribed. For *hyperkalemia,* provide diet low in potassium and instruct the patient regarding the presence of K⁺ in food; administer Kayexalate orally or rectally. For *hypokalemia,* administer potassium supplements as prescribed; instruct the patient regarding foods high in potassium.

4. Monitor the patient receiving digoxin for toxicity (anorexia, nausea, vomiting, diarrhea, and seeing halos around objects). Monitor the ECG for bigeminy or premature ventricular contractions.

5. Monitor the acid–base balance.

6. If hyperkalemia worsens, institute the nursing management outlined in Table 48–9 related to hyperkalemia.

---

1. *Hyperkalemia* may result from altered excretory mechanisms of the tubule, excessive tissue damage, GI bleeding, transfusions of stored blood, large hematomas, administration of potassium-sparing diuretics, or excessive administration of potassium. *Hypokalemia* may result from tubular defects, use of potassium-losing diuretics, and diarrhea.

2. Potassium imbalances alter the resting potential of muscle cells.

3. Frequently, potassium imbalances can be corrected by proper diet and/or use of oral medications. Foods high in potassium include fruits, meat, milk, white potatoes, and legumes.

4. Hypokalemia potentiates the effect of digoxin. In addition, digoxin is excreted by the kidneys, so requirements of the drug are less in patients with renal insufficiency and failure.

5. Hyperkalemia and metabolic acidosis are intimately related. In severe metabolic acidosis, hydrogen ions move into the cells and K⁺ ions move into the interstitial fluid and blood, thus causing hyperkalemia. Hypokalemia and metabolic alkalosis are also related.

6. The patient needs to be carefully monitored because the level of K⁺ may be unstable.

C. Problems in Maintenance of a Normal Urine Output

Problems Related to Decreased Urine Output

1. Monitor the urine:
   - Measure the volume.
   - Measure the specific gravity.
   - Note the color.

2. Administer oral and parenteral fluids as prescribed.

3. If fluids are restricted, provide meticulous oral hygiene at least three times a day.

4. Monitor the vital signs and breath and heart sounds, and note the presence of edema; the frequency depends on the condition of the patient. Consult with the physician about abnormal findings.

5. Teach the patient the reason for the fluid restriction. State the amount of fluid allowed in a 24-hour period and plan the intake with the patient.

6. Maintain accurate records of intake, output, and weight, and compare the findings (1 kg [2.2 lb] represents 1,000 mL fluid).

7. Consult with the physician about any significant changes in the patient's cardiovascular status or in the laboratory studies that may indicate a deterioration of kidney function.

---

1. A decreased urine output may result from (a) a decreased number of functioning nephrons, leading to water retention or (b) decreased renal perfusion from hypovolemia. The urine volume is decreased and specific gravity is increased in hypovolemia.

2. The amount of fluid restriction required will depend on the volume status.

3. Proper oral hygiene assists in relieving thirst.

4. Fluid retention can cause hypervolemia. If excessive, heart failure and pulmonary edema can result. Noting the early signs of heart failure and initiating treatment early can prevent serious complications.

5. The ability to urinate has a strong psychologic significance. When this function is altered, the patient may feel out of control. By being included in the planning, the patient may be able to recover some of this control and feel better about himself or herself and be more compliant with restrictions.

6. These records are essential in determining fluid status. Increased intake and weight with a decreased urinary output can precipitate heart failure.

7. Significant changes may require alterations in the mode of treatment. The nurse needs to determine if the alteration needs immediate attention (i.e., presence of hyperkalemia, which may cause lethal arrhythmias) or if the alteration simply needs follow-up evaluation (i.e., small decrease in hemoglobin).

(Continued)

TABLE 47–7 *(Continued)*

NURSING MANAGEMENT PLAN: THE PATIENT WITH RENAL INSUFFICIENCY

Interventions	Rationale/Significance
Problem With Excessive Urine Production	
1. Monitor the patient for volume depletion. Monitor signs of inability to concentrate the urine, which include polyuria, nocturia, large volumes of pale urine, and thirst.	1. A large amount of dilute urine may be excreted when nephrons hypertrophy, in acute renal failure, or in tubular disorders.
2. Monitor the specific gravity of the urine.	2. The specific gravity will be less than 1.010 in dilute urine.
3. See Chap. 8 for additional nursing management related to hypovolemia.	3. This patient has to be monitored carefully to prevent hypovolemia.
D. Problems Related to Protein and Blood in the Urine	
Proteinuria	
1. Assist in preventing protein malnutrition.	1. Protein malnutrition may result from massive proteinuria as typically seen in the nephrotic syndrome.
a. Provide the prescribed diet.	a. Proteins with high biologic value should be used for replacement of proteins lost in urine. Although traditionally a high-protein diet has been prescribed, many physicians now recommend a *low-protein* diet. It is believed that this decreases filtration of protein across the glomerular membrane and thus helps prevent further renal damage.
b. Administer prescribed albumin IV.	b. Albumin is the protein most commonly lost in glomerular disease.
2. Monitor serum total protein and serum albumin values and urinary protein values.	2. Low serum total protein and serum albumin and high urinary protein indicate protein malnutrition.
3. Encourage the patient to avoid fatigue.	3. Many of these patients do not feel "well" and have decreased endurance and tolerance to activity.
Hematuria	
1. Identify hematuria. Record the degree of hematuria by inspecting the color of the urine and by using a hemastix that classifies the degree of hematuria from negative to large amounts.	1. Blood is not a normal constituent of urine.
2. Monitor the hemoglobin and hematocrit values.	2. Low hemoglobin and hematocrit values may indicate anemia or hypervolemic dilution.
3. Monitor the patient for tachycardia, pale skin and conjunctivae, dizziness, chest pain, dyspnea, and weakness.	3. Anemia is diagnosed on the basis of laboratory studies as well as the presenting symptoms.
4. Recognize possible causes of hematuria.	4. Hematuria may occur with chronic glomerulonephritis, nephrolithiasis, cystitis, urinary tract trauma, and reactions to blood transfusions.
a. Monitor the patient for pain that may begin in the costovertebral angle or the flank and may migrate toward the groin.	a. Hematuria per se is asymptomatic but it may be accompanied by renal colic (ureteral spasms produced by the irritation of a stone or blood clot and accompanying obstruction). Patients with renal stones may be asymptomatic or may have severe pain.
b. Note diagnostic tests that may cause hematuria.	b. Hematuria may be normal following a renal biopsy, but must be monitored closely. It may also follow urinary catheterization or other instrumentation.
c. Review medications being taken that may cause hematuria.	c. If the patient is receiving anticoagulants, hematuria may be an adverse reaction indicating (1) coagulation abnormalities or (2) the need to decrease the dose.
d. Review the patient's history and reason for current hospitalization.	d. Hematuria following a motor vehicle accident indicates trauma to the urinary tract. Cystic kidney disease and malignancy are frequently manifested by hematuria.

Interventions	**Rationale/Significance**

E. Problems With Preserving Renal Function

1. Teach the patient and the family about the patient's specific disease and the symptoms to report (i.e., occurrence of or increased edema, dyspnea, nausea, vomiting, anorexia, lethargy, and decreased urinary output).

2. Monitor and compare BUN and creatinine results in patients receiving nephrotoxic drugs, such as aminoglycoside antibiotics, or patients in shock. Confer with the physician about a significant report that he or she has not had an opportunity to see.

3. Maintain optimum hydration, unless contraindicated.

4. Monitor the patient closely during administration of blood transfusions. If there are signs of a reaction (chills, sudden changes in vital signs, and hematuria), implement the care plan related to blood transfusions in Chap. 28.

F. Problems With Increased Susceptibility to Infection

1. Monitor all vital signs closely. Observe for tachycardia, tachypnea, changes in temperature, and hypotension.

2. Monitor the white blood count and differential.

3. If hospitalized, limit visitation to noninfectious individuals and minimize contact with other patients with infections. In the community, teach the patient to avoid exposure to those who are ill and to avoid crowds during epidemics of influenza and colds. In the hospital, avoid assigning the patient to a staff member who has a cold or who is taking care of another patient in isolation.

4. When possible, avoid the use of indwelling catheters.

5. When catheterization is necessary, provide routine periurethral care every 8 hours.

6. Always maintain a downward flow of urine to the collection bag.

7. Use meticulous handwashing technique before and after intravenous care.

8. Assist in identifying organisms responsible for infection:
   - Routinely inspect all potential sites for infection: IV sites, surgical wounds, traumatized areas, decubitus ulcers, and secretions from tracheostomies.
   - Use appropriate senses of sight (redness, swelling) smell, and touch (warmth) to assist in determining if an infection is present. Use adequate light.
   - Obtain cultures of suspected infectious sites (by prescription or by institutional policy related to infection control). Chart the sites where specimens are obtained. Report suspected infectious sites to the physician.

9. Cleanse the urethral meatus well prior to collecting a urine specimen for analysis.

Rationale/Significance

1. Increased knowledge may foster increased compliance with the treatment regimen.

2. A rise in the serum BUN and creatinine levels is significant, indicating that renal function is deteriorating because the kidneys are losing their ability to remove these waste products. If the levels rise, the physician has to weigh the risks and advantages in the continued use or discontinuance of the aminoglycoside for each patient.

3. Hypovolemia may result in hypotension, which can lead to decreased blood supply to the kidney and possibly to acute tubular necrosis (ATN).

4. Mismatched blood may cause necrosis of the tubules and further nephron loss.

1. Body temperature is often misleading; patients with kidney disease may have a low body temperature even with an infection.

2. The increase in the white blood count in response to infection may be less than usual in patients with kidney disease. An increase in polymorphonuclear neutrophils occurs with the onset of acute infection.

3. Increased susceptibility to infection may be caused by urinary loss of plasma proteins, which contain antibodies, or by the presence of uremia, which predisposes the patient to infection. Avoiding pathogens in the environment decreases the risk of infection.

4. Indwelling catheters are an excellent route of infection to the bladder, then to the kidneys.

5. Proper cleansing of the periurethral area decreases the microbial population and lessens the chance of organisms ascending the catheter and causing infection.

6. Although urine is sterile and the collection bag is sterile when it is first attached, the bag has the potential for becoming contaminated with repeated emptying. Therefore, the bag is not considered to be sterile once it is hung.

7. Minimizing the bacterial population on your hands prevents the hematogenous introduction of organisms that may infect the kidneys.

8. By including an "infection assessment" in the daily care of the patient, potential infections may be quickly identified and treatment begun.

9. Cleansing the meatus adequately will prevent contamination of the urine from bacteria at the distal urethra.

(Continued)

TABLE 47–7   *(Continued)*

NURSING MANAGEMENT PLAN: THE PATIENT WITH RENAL INSUFFICIENCY

Interventions	Rationale/Significance
10. Refrigerate urine specimen if it cannot be cultured immediately.	10. Refrigeration will inhibit growth of all bacteria.
11. Administer prescribed antibiotics promptly and carefully.	11. By reducing the bacterial population of the urinary tract with antibiotics, progressive renal damage may be prevented.
12. Once a site has been cultured, review all sensitivity reports. Note whether the patient is receiving antibiotics to which the organisms that are present are sensitive. If not, confer with the physician.	12. Frequently physicians will prescribe a broad-spectrum antibiotic as initial therapy until the results of the culture are available. If the identified organism is not sensitive to this antibiotic, the physician will usually discontinue it and prescribe one to which the organism is sensitive.
13. Teach the patient to maintain an adequate diet and to allow time for rest.	13. Optimal health status increases the ability of the body to fight infection.
G. Problems Affecting the Skin	
1. Monitor the skin periodically for changes in color, turgor, texture, and vascularity.	1. The skin may be a grayish-bronze color from the retention of deposits of lipid-soluble pigments. Pallor may indicate anemia. Alterations in texture may result from dehydration. Increased capillary fragility may cause purpura.
2. Keep the skin clean and aid in relieving itching and dryness using one of the following methods: basic soap, bath oil, oatmeal baths, sodium bicarbonate in bath water, or a lanolin base lotion.	2. There may be a decrease in the activity of oil glands and size of sweat glands.
3. Monitor serum phosphate levels and serum calcium levels.	3. Pruritus may occur because of the presence of phosphate (PO_4) crystal deposits in the skin. Serum phosphate levels increase because of the kidney's inability to remove PO_4 from the body. As the serum PO_4 increases, the serum Ca will decrease.
4. In the patient with edema, inspect the patient's skin over the extremities, back, and buttocks (especially the bony prominences) for breakdown.	4. A compromised circulatory system and edema may result in decubitus ulcers. Red areas may indicate pressure points that are most vulnerable to skin breakdown.
5. Encourage the patient to turn at least every 2 hours and maintain a position that relieves the pressure over these areas; assist as necessary. Massage vulnerable areas gently. Apply an egg crate mattress or sheep skin to the bed.	5. Relieving pressure from vulnerable areas increases circulation and cellular nutrition.
6. Apply prescribed antiembolism stockings. Measure the lower extremities when obtaining stockings to ensure a proper fit.	6. Antiembolism stockings promote circulation from the superficial veins to the deep veins in edematous legs.
7. Encourage active range-of-motion exercises or, if necessary, provide passive range-of-motion exercises.	7. Exercises improve circulation.

propriate actions to limit susceptibility to infection, and care for the skin to prevent breakdown

The patient on immunosuppressive therapy will:

5. Maintain an exercise program, select a diet with limited simple carbohydrates such as sugars, maintain good skin hygiene, and take medications as prescribed

CARE OF PATIENTS NEEDING URETHRAL CATHETERIZATION

Urethral catheterization refers to the insertion of a catheter through the urethra into the bladder. Intermittent catheterization is performed either to drain the urine when the patient is unable to void normally or to obtain a urine speci-

men for diagnostic data. An indwelling Foley catheter is used for continuous catheterization when the patient cannot void or is incontinent (when other measures are not effective) or the output must be closely monitored.

Because catheterization involves touching the genitalia, particular effort is made to preserve the patient's dignity during the procedure. Privacy is provided, and unnecessary exposure is avoided.

Nosocomial, or hospital-acquired, infections affect at least 2 million of the 40 million patients hospitalized annually in the United States. *Urinary tract infections are the leading cause of these infections, estimated at 40%.* It is estimated that nosocomial infections contribute directly to at least 50,000 deaths annually; they also add 15 million extra days of hospitalization at a cost of over 5 billion dollars annually.[73]

TABLE 47-8

NURSING MANAGEMENT PLAN: THE PATIENT WITH POTENTIAL PROBLEMS RELATED TO CORTICOSTEROID/IMMUNOSUPPRESSANT THERAPY

Potential Nursing Diagnoses/Collaborative Problems
- *Protection, altered, related to drug therapy to depress the immune system*
- *Fluid volume excess related to adverse effects of immunosuppressant drugs*
- *Body image disturbance related to adverse effects of immunosuppressant drugs*
- *Knowledge deficit related to drug therapy and diet*

Goals/Desired Outcomes
- *The patient will (a) maintain muscle tone and fluid and electrolyte balance, (b) eat the prescribed diet, (c) maintain self-care measures, (d) take prescribed medicines, and (e) avoid complications.*

Interventions	Rationale/Significance
Corticosteroid Therapy	
1. Monitor the patient for centripetal weight gain (weight gain primarily in the torso). Encourage exercise to retain muscle tone. Emphasize strict adherence to a diet with decreased carbohydrates, especially sugar. Monitor the blood sugar.	1. Excessive weight gain is due to voracious appetite. Carbohydrate intolerance occurs with steroids. Steroid-dependent diabetes may develop.
2. Monitor for hirsutism of the face, trunk, and extremities. Tell the patient that the hair can be bleached, shaved, or removed with a depilatory cream.	2. Hirsutism is related to the androgenic effect of steroids.
3. Monitor for alopecia. Inform the patient that the usual hair growth will return. Encourage the use of a wig or toupee.	3. Alopecia is also related to the androgenic effect of steroids.
4. Monitor for ecchymoses, petechiae, purpura, and gingival bleeding. Encourage a diet high in protein (*if allowed*) and vitamin C. Avoid venipunctures, which can cause subcutaneous hemorrhage. Monitor platelet counts for thrombocytopenia. Encourage use of a soft toothbrush.	4. Capillary fragility and low platelet counts account for these clinical findings.
5. Monitor for acne. Teach the importance of good personal hygiene with soap and water. Advise to avoid oily lotions.	5. Papules and pustules are common.
6. Monitor for thinning of the skin. Avoid the use of adhesive tape. Aid in preventing decubitus formation by encouraging the patient to change positions frequently. Caution against sunburn.	6. Thin skin is extremely susceptible to breakdown.
7. Monitor fluid and electrolyte balance closely. Monitor blood pressure closely. Assess for edema in the feet, fingers, eyelids, and sacrum (and in the scrotum in the male patient). Monitor for signs of heart failure and pulmonary edema (tachycardia, tachypnea, crackles, and rhonchi). Weigh correctly daily. Maintain prescribed fluid restriction. Administer prescribed diuretic drug therapy.	7. Sodium (and thus water) is retained and potassium lost because of the increased levels of corticosteroids. Hypertension may develop as a result of sodium and water retention.
8. Monitor for major signs of cancer.	8. There is increased incidence or recurrence of malignancies of the epithelial tissues and deep tumors because of the inhibition of the immune surveillance mechanism.
9. Provide psychologic support. Monitor the mental status. Explain that mood swings are common.	9. Changes in physical appearance (moon facies, fat redistribution) are often very distressing for patients. Psychosis can occur as an untoward effect.

10. Monitor for GI bleeding.
  • Check all stools for gross blood.
  • Check vomitus for gross blood.
  • Monitor the hemoglobin and hematocrit levels.
  • Ask about epigastric discomfort.
  • Encourage frequent and regular meals.
  • Administer prescribed antacids with steroids and when the stomach is empty (2 hours pc and hs).
  • Administer a prescribed histamine H_2 antagonist (cimetidine [Tagamet] or ranitidine [Zantac]) to inhibit hydrochloric acid production.
	10. GI irritation is due to increased hydrochloric acid production and changes in the GI mucosa.

(Continued)

TABLE 47–8   (*Continued*)

NURSING MANAGEMENT PLAN: THE PATIENT WITH POTENTIAL PROBLEMS RELATED TO CORTICOSTEROID/IMMUNOSUPPRESSANT THERAPY

Interventions	Rationale/Significance
11. Monitor closely for signs and symptoms of infection. (See previous care plan.)	11. Steroids mask signs and symptoms of infection. A slight increase in temperature (greater than 99°F) is significant.
Immunosuppressive Therapy	
1. Monitor serum creatinine and BUN. Emphasize the importance of periodic laboratory tests to monitor kidney function.	1. Drugs like cyclosporine are nephrotoxic and can cause a reduction in renal function.
2. Monitor for early signs of infection (fever, sore throat) and report immediately to the physician.	2. Bone marrow suppression may lead to leukopenia.

(Sources: *Lehne et al,*[41] *O'Donnell.*[55])

Types of Catheters

Many different catheters are available for special purposes. Figure 47–11 illustrates a few of these types.

1. A *round-tip* (also called a *Robinson, plain,* or *straight*) *catheter* is a soft synthetic rubber or plastic catheter with a rounded end and one or two openings (eyes) on the sides of the distal portion.

2. The *whistle-tip catheter* is similar to the round-tip catheter, but the terminal opening is cut obliquely across the end. It is ideal for use when hematuria and blood clots are present.

3. A *Pezzer* ("*mushroom*") *catheter* is a single-channel self-retaining catheter with a mushroom-shaped tip. A stylet that straightens the tip is used during insertion and removal. It is rarely passed through the urethra. It is usually inserted through a surgically made suprapubic opening into the bladder or used as a nephrostomy tube in the renal pelvis.

4. A *Malecot catheter* is a two-winged or four-winged single-channeled self-retaining catheter. It has the same uses and methods of insertion and removal as the Pezzer catheter.

5. A *Foley, double-lumen catheter* is any type of catheter with an inflatable balloon near the distal tip. The inflated balloon (holds 5 to 30 mL solution for adults) holds the catheter indwelling. It can be used as a cystostomy tube for an opening into the bladder.

6. A *Foley, triple-lumen catheter* has a balloon plus lumens for drainage and irrigation of the bladder.

7. A *coudé curved-tip catheter* should be used if catheterization of the male urethra is difficult; it is more easily passed in the angulation between the bulbous and membranous urethra.

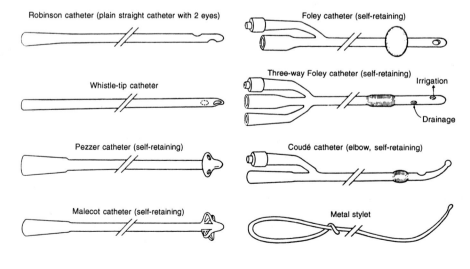

Figure 47–11. Urethral catheters and a metal stylet that is used for insertion and removal of self-retaining catheters. (*From Tanagho and McAninch.*[79])

Urethral catheters are labeled according to the size of the lumen, using French units, which approximately correspond to 0.33 mm in diameter (18 French denotes a diameter of 6 mm). Sizes commonly used for the adult female and male are sizes 14 and 16 French. The smallest indwelling catheter should be selected that will drain the bladder, because it also allows periurethral tissues to drain secretions, such as mucus, around the outer lumen.

Nursing Management of the Patient With an Indwelling Catheter

Urethral catheterization should be considered an invasive procedure. Nurses have primary responsibility for insertion of catheters and care of indwelling catheters. Nurses should be knowledgeable about the importance of utilizing and maintaining aseptic technique and the recognition and prevention of complications. They should use every opportunity to teach nonprofessional caregivers as well as patients about proper catheter care. Table 47–9 summarizes the care of a patient with an indwelling catheter. Aspects of the catheterization procedure are also discussed. The technical aspects of insertion, daily care, observation, and supportive care must be thoroughly understood for excellent patient care. Infection can be introduced in multiple ways, so adhering to aseptic technique when caring for these catheters is vital in reducing the possibility of infection in these patients.

Shock and Urine Drainage

For years it has been standard practice not to remove more than 1,000 mL of urine at one time; the catheter is clamped for 30 minutes, and then additional urine is drained. Removing more than this amount has been thought to release pressure on pelvic blood vessels and lead to shock.

A *research study* was done of ten males with acute urinary retention. The intravesical pressure and blood pressure were recorded during either continuous drainage in seven males or fractionated drainage in three males. After removal of the initial 100 mL urine, the intravesical pressure declined to approximately 50% of the initial pressure in both groups; pain was relieved in all patients when this amount was removed. The amount of urine that was drained ranged from 450 to 3,100 mL. The blood pressure was lowered in all patients with a median before drainage of 117.5 mm Hg and a median after drainage of 109 mm Hg. This decrease was significant ($p < .05$), but none of the patients developed any clinical symptoms of hypotension. The researchers concluded that there is no support for the recommendation of fractionated bladder drainage.[15]

Care of the Patient After Urethral Catheter Removal

Bladder dysfunction following prolonged catheterization is a major problem for many patients. The patient may have problems with bacteriuria, mucosal irritation, or bladder distention and retention of residual urine as a result of incomplete bladder emptying during voiding. Normally the bladder is almost completely emptied at each micturition. The bladder wall is made of transitional muscle that is able to expand and contract. Constant drainage of urine from the bladder by an indwelling catheter keeps the detrusor muscle in a state of continual constriction. This prolonged disuse of the bladder muscle influences tone, making the muscle weak from lack of exercise.

The patient is encouraged to maintain a high fluid intake, if not contraindicated, and to empty the bladder as soon as the urge to void is present. Bladder dysfunction seems to diminish with each micturition after catheter removal. The patient's bladder is assessed by palpation and percussion, the voiding status is monitored, and the patient is assessed for signs of urinary tract infection.

Clean Intermittent Self-catheterization

An important step in rehabilitation of a patient with a neurogenic bladder or some other cause of incontinence requiring catheterization is developing the ability to meet daily hygienic needs. Intermittent self-catheterization is one way this goal may be met. Intermittent urinary catheterization has been advocated as the preferred method to artificially empty the bladder that retains or does not completely release urine. When compared with the indwelling catheter, the use of intermittent catheterization reportedly promotes an earlier return of bladder functioning while reducing the incidence of urinary tract infections.[70] Intermittent catheterization is preferred to indwelling catheterization because it allows the bladder to fill normally; simulates normal voiding; provides a means of expelling urine, including residual urine; avoids incontinence; and helps prevent infection.

A structured teaching program must be developed to provide information necessary for the patient to learn the technique of self-catheterization. The program includes (1) normal anatomy of the urinary system, (2) purpose of the catheterization, and (3) a thorough explanation of clean technique. The patient is told that sterile technique is required while hospitalized because of the danger of infection from other patients or staff members, but clean technique can be used after return to the home. The patient continues to perform the procedure under direct nursing supervision before discharge until he or she feels completely comfortable with each step. The female patient may need to use a mirror propped between her legs to locate the meatus. A device called "female self-cath aide" can be custom made by the occupational therapist. It is designed with a tampon-like projection that fits into the vagina so that a "funnel" fits directly over the urinary meatus to allow for ease in introducing a catheter.[87]

The importance of maintaining a daily catheterization routine to prevent overdistention of the bladder is stressed. Overdistention can lead to a compromised blood supply to the mucosa due to pressure on the mucosal vessels. Stasis of urine in the bladder may also lead to infection. The recommended frequency of catheterization varies; most patients benefit from intermittent drainage every 3 to 6 hours. A patient who drinks 1.5 to 2 L should catheterize four to five times per day (at equal time intervals) during the waking hours. Bladder volumes of approximately 360 mL (12 oz) are best for maintaining good bladder function. In

TABLE 47-9

NURSING MANAGEMENT PLAN: THE PATIENT REQUIRING AN INDWELLING URINARY CATHETER

Potential Nursing Diagnoses/Collaborative Problems
- *Protection, altered, related to the potential for introducing pathogens into the urinary tract*
- *Urinary elimination, altered, related to urinary incontinence, obstruction, or retention*
- *Knowledge deficit related to principles of catheter care*

Goals/Desired Outcomes
- *The patient will experience minimal discomfort during insertion and while the indwelling catheter is in place and will develop no complications.*

Interventions	Rationale/Significance
Care Prior to Catheterization	
1. Inform the patient about the purpose of the catheterization, general steps of the procedure, how the patient can cooperate during the procedure, and what symptoms to report. Explain that the procedure should not be painful but that a sensation of pressure or burning may be felt. Explain that a cold, wet feeling will be experienced when the cleansing solutions are used. State that taking slow, deep breaths may help him or her to relax.	1. Providing information may lessen the patient's anxiety.
2. Gather the equipment: catheterization tray (select the smallest functional catheter) with drainage system. Wash your hands.	2. Prepackaged sterile catheterization trays and drainage systems are available.
3. Ensure privacy by screening the patient and placing a sign stating "No admittance—procedure in progress" on the door. Assist the patient to lie supine with the legs bent and spread apart. Prevent coolness by covering the patient's upper body and the feet with blankets, if needed.	3. Coolness causes muscle tension and lessens the ability to maintain proper positioning.
Care During Catheterization of the Female Patient	
1. Don nonsterile gloves to examine the perineal area to determine if the urethral meatus is readily seen. If not, have a sterile applicator placed on the sterile field in the catheter tray prior to catheterization.	1. Prior to catheterization, the applicator can be placed in the vagina to aid in determining landmarks.
2. After placing the tray between the patient's legs, open the wrapper and spread it to form a sterile field. Remove waterproof underpad from tray and place under the patient's hips, while maintaining a sterile field. Don the sterile gloves. Place the fenestrated drape with hole in center over the perineal area. If needed, ask assistant to place a sterile cotton-tipped applicator on the sterile field.	2. Sterile technique is maintained while the drapes are placed.
3. Remove one cotton ball from tray of cotton balls. Open cleansing solution and pour it over the cotton balls.	3. The dry cotton ball is used to remove excess cleansing solution.
4. Inflate the balloon with appropriate amount of sterile water, then withdraw the solution. Attach the catheter to the drainage collection system. Close the drainage spout.	4. It is best to test the balloon prior to insertion to be certain that it is functioning correctly. The balloon is inflated with 8 to 9 mL sterile water. The balloon holds 5 mL; the extra 3 to 4 mL will fill the lumen leading to the balloon.
5. Lubricate the distal 2 in. of the catheter generously with available water-soluble lubricant.	5. Lubricant lessens the friction between the catheter and urethral mucosa as the catheter is being inserted.
6. With nondominant hand, spread the labia apart and gently pull the tissue upward to smooth out the perineum and assist in visualizing the meatus. Maintain this position throughout the insertion. If needed, ask an assistant to shine a light over the perineal area. If needed, place a cotton-tipped applicator in the vagina. Grasp forceps on tray with dominant hand, then use individual cotton balls to cleanse the urethral meatus. Take single downward stroke with each ball over each labia minora, then centrally over the urethral meatus last. Blot meatus with a dry cotton ball.	6. Visualizing the meatus well and determining the correct place to insert the catheter can lessen trauma.

Interventions	Rationale/Significance
7. Gently insert the lubricated end of the catheter into the meatus until urine begins to flow. *Do not* force the catheter.	7. Force can damage the urethra.
8. Insert the catheter about another 1 to 2 in., and then inflate the balloon with 8 to 9 mL of sterile water. Observe the patient during balloon inflation. If there are complaints of pain, withdraw all of the solution, advance the catheter ½ in., then inflate the balloon again. Gently tug on the catheter to check that the balloon is anchoring the catheter in the bladder.	8. Further insertion ensures that the balloon portion is in the bladder rather than the urethra.
9. Use soap and water to remove the cleansing solution from the perineal area.	9. These solutions can be irritating to the skin.
10. Remove gloves and anchor the catheter to the upper aspect of the patient's thigh (Fig. 47–12A). Leave slack in the catheter to prevent pull on the catheter when the leg is moved.	10. The catheter is anchored to avoid unnecessary strain on the trigone of the bladder and to prevent the catheter from moving in and out of the bladder, which could cause inflammation from friction. Some physicians request that the catheter be taped to the patient's abdomen to lessen the likelihood of migration of enteric bacteria from the anus.
11. Place the drainage tubing over the top of the thigh. Secure the drainage tube to the sheet, leaving enough slack so that the patient can turn. Loop extra tubing on the bed.	11. Urine can flow better when there are no dependent loops in the tubing.
12. Secure the drainage bag to the bed frame, *not* to the side rails.	12. Tension may be placed on the bag when the side rails are raised or lowered, thereby possibly pulling on the catheter within the patient's bladder.
13. Discard contents appropriately. Wash your hands. Attach a piece of tape to the tubing stating the date the catheter is inserted and by whom. Record time, size of catheter inserted, and any untoward effects experienced by the patient.	13. Documentation is important.

Care During Catheterization of the Male Patient

Interventions	Rationale/Significance
1. Implement steps 1–3 of the Care Prior to Catheterization.	1. The preliminary care is the same.
2. After placing the tray between the patient's legs, open the wrapper and spread it to form a sterile field. Remove waterproof underpad from tray and place under the patient's hips, while maintaining a sterile field. Don the sterile gloves. Place the second drape with hole in center over the penis.	2. Sterile technique is maintained while the drapes are placed.
3. Remove one cotton ball from tray of cotton balls. Open cleansing solution and pour it over the cotton balls.	3. The dry cotton ball is used to remove excess cleansing solution.
4. Inflate the balloon with appropriate amount of sterile water to test balloon function, then withdraw the solution. Attach the catheter to the drainage collection system. Close the drainage spout.	4. It is best to test the balloon prior to insertion to be certain that it is functioning correctly.
5. Lubricate the catheter to the bifurcation (Y) with available water-soluble lubricant.	5. Lubricant lessens the friction between the catheter and urethral mucosa as the catheter is being inserted.
6. With nondominant hand, hold the patient's penis taut. If the patient is uncircumcised, pull the foreskin back with the same hand. Grasp forceps on tray with dominant hand, and then use individual cotton balls to cleanse the urethral meatus. Clean the meatus using a circular motion from the meatus outward and continue in a circular motion by cleaning 2 to 3 in. down the shaft. Blot meatus and shaft with dry cotton ball.	6. Light stimulation may cause an erection. If this does occur, the procedure is discontinued, the patient is informed that the procedure will be delayed until the erection subsides, the patient is covered, and the nurse leaves the room for a few minutes.
7. Hold the penis at a 90-degree angle to the patient's thighs. Gently insert the lubricated end of the catheter into the meatus. Lower the penis to a 60-degree angle. Using gentle but steady pressure, insert the catheter to the bifurcation (Y) of the catheter. *If strong resistance is felt, do not force the catheter.* Withdraw it and notify the physician.	7. When the increased resistance of the prostatic urethra is encountered, the penis is lowered. The entire length of the catheter should be passed so that the balloon is not in the urethra when it is inflated.

(Continued)

TABLE 47-9   *(Continued)*

NURSING MANAGEMENT PLAN: THE PATIENT REQUIRING AN INDWELLING URINARY CATHETER

Interventions	Rationale/Significance
8. After the catheter is inserted, inflate the balloon with the appropriate amount of solution. Gently tug on the catheter to check that the balloon is anchoring the catheter in the bladder. In the uncircumcised patient, pull foreskin back to its normal position.	8. Further insertion ensures that the balloon portion is in the bladder rather than the urethra.
9. Use soap and water to remove the cleansing solution.	9. These solutions can be irritating to the skin.
10. Remove gloves and anchor the catheter to the patient's abdomen (Fig. 47–12B). Leave slack in the catheter so that traction is not produced.	10. The penis is not left in its usual position after an indwelling catheter is inserted. The penoscrotal angle may be compressed because of the tendency of the catheter to straighten. An abscess or a pressure sore can form, which can subsequently develop into a urethrocutaneous fistula.
11. Implement steps 11–13 of Care During Catheterization of the Female Patient.	11. These steps are the same for males and females.

Care While Indwelling Catheter Is in Place

1. Clean around the meatal–catheter junction using a bath cloth, soap, and water at least twice daily. Begin at the meatus and gently proceed distally on the catheter for several inches. Remove any encrustations from the outside of the catheter. Dry the area well.	1. Microorganisms can migrate up the external portion of the catheter. Cleansing reduces the number of microorganisms and removes encrustations.
2. Follow the protocol for your institution about application of ointment around the meatal–catheter junction. If used, apply with a sterile applicator.	2. Some institutions use only soap and water, with the rationale that the ointment may harbor bacteria. Others state to apply a lubricating ointment or an antibiotic or iodine (Betadine) ointment.
3. Wear gloves. Always wash your hands carefully before and after contact with the catheter or drainage bag.	3. Handwashing and gloving are necessary to prevent cross-contamination and for protection of the nurse.
4a. Do not disconnect the catheter or drainage tubing once it is attached.	4a. Disconnecting the system breaks the sterility of the system.
b. Empty the drainage bag at least every 8 hours. Do not allow the tip of the drain to touch the collection container. Cleanse the tip of the drain with an alcohol sponge after draining the urine, and then tuck it in its cover.	b. Cleansing the drain after draining the urine removes urine that may be present and lessens the chance of bacterial growth on the drain.
5. Observe the tubing for kinks or obstruction. If the tubing is occluded, milk the tubing *toward* the drainage bag to try to dislodge the obstructing particles. If irrigation is necessary, use sterile technique while irrigating the catheter with sterile saline or a prescribed solution. If none of these measures is effective, consult with the physican.	5. If the entire tube is filled with urine, it may be obstructed.
6. Maintain the drainage bag below the level of the bladder. Do not allow the bag to touch the floor.	6. When the bag is higher than the bladder, urine may flow from the tubing back into the bladder, increasing the chance of infection.
7. Monitor the patient for bacteriuria: persistent burning at the catheter site, cloudy urine, or odorous urine.	7. Bacteriuria is common with an indwelling catheter.
8. Monitor the drainage bag and the catheter to determine when they need to be changed. Roll the distal end of the catheter between your fingers. Change the catheter if sandy particles are felt. Change the drainage bag if it leaks, if it becomes odorous, if the catheter is changed, or in accordance with institutional protocols. In addition to charting the information, attach a piece of tape to the tubing stating the date the catheter and bag were changed and by whom.	8. It is important to document when the catheter and drainage systems are changed.
9. Encourage the patient to increase fluid intake to 3 L unless contraindicated by renal or cardiac disease.	9. This increases the urinary output and may lessen the possibility of a urinary tract infection.
10. Encourage the patient to turn from side to back to side.	10. This promotes drainage.

(Sources: *Smith,*[67] *Smith and Duell.*[68])

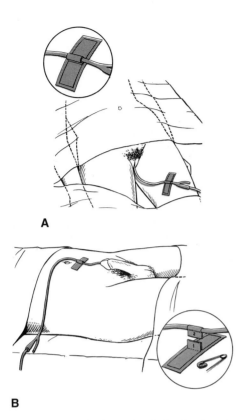

A

B

Figure 47–12. Taping of urethral catheters. **A.** For *female,* catheter can be secured to thigh with two strips of tape. *Inset:* Place first strip of tape on thigh. Place center of second strip of tape around catheter, then attach ends of strip to first tape strip. **B.** For *male,* catheter is secured to abdomen below navel using three strips of tape. *Inset:* Place first tape strip on abdomen. Form tab 1 with second tape strip and attach to first strip. Form tab 2 around catheter with third tape strip. Pin the two tabs together. (*From Norton and Miller.*[34])

TABLE 47–10

TEACHING PLAN: THE PATIENT REQUIRING CLEAN INTERMITTENT SELF-CATHETERIZATION

1. Remember that washing your hands or using a disposable towelette before each catheterization is very important.
2. A sterilizing solution is not necessary to cleanse the perineum or end of the penis; no lubricant is needed for the female patient.
3. Remember that *regular* catheterization is extremely important.
4. For the *female* patient, learn how to palpate the meatus. With the left hand (those who are left-handed should reverse all references) hold the labia apart with the index and ring fingers and palpate the urethra with the middle finger. You will eventually perform the procedure entirely by touch so that a mirror will not be necessary. Learn to hold the catheter in the right hand between the thumb and forefinger and insert it into the meatus. The distal end of the catheter is held over the basin.
5. For the *male* patient, grasp the penis with the left hand and simultaneously insert the catheter into the meatus, while extending the penis upward and toward the umbilicus (in a "J" position), and on into the bladder.
6. Assess the urine drainage for any abnormal constituents (blood, sediment, odor, or cloudiness). Note any discomfort (back or abdominal), evidence of fever, or trouble passing the catheter. Notify the health care professional if any of these signs are present.
7. Drink cranberry or prune juice to maintain an acid urine pH.
8. After the procedure is completed, wash the inside and outside of the catheter with soapy water, then rinse it. Shake the catheter to remove most of the water from the inside, dry the outside, then store it in a clean container.

(Sources: *Kozier et al,*[39] *Smith,*[67] *Weber-Jones.*[87])

order to achieve a full night's sleep, the patient should catheterize immediately before retiring. The patient should be cautioned to consume the majority of fluids by the evening meal and to avoid drinking fluids at least 3 hours prior to bedtime.[87] The schedule for catheterization is individualized to prevent infection, bladder overdistention and incontinence, and damage to the upper urinary tract. Infections as the result of intermittent catheterization are infrequent, but may be treated with once-daily prophylactic antibiotics.[80] The patient should be encouraged to drink cranberry or prune juice to maintain an acid urine pH that will retard the risk of infection.

The patient is taught how to record information concerning the time of catheterization and amount, color, and odor of urine obtained. The patient should contact the health care professional about problems encountered during the procedure and between catheterizations. The points in the teaching plan in Table 47–10 need to be emphasized.

Evaluation/Desired Outcomes. The patient:

1. Requiring intermittent catheterization will recover the ability to void and will not develop a urinary tract infection

2. Requiring an indwelling catheter will not develop a urinary tract infection and will drink sufficient fluids to increase the urinary output
3. Requiring clean, intermittent self-catheterization will perform the procedure correctly

CARE OF PATIENTS WITH URINARY INCONTINENCE

Incontinence is a general term referring to the involuntary loss of urine. Studies have shown that many individuals will experience some degree of incontinence during their lifetimes and that women are more prone to incontinence than men. A *research study* indicates that, after 35 years of age, more than 10% of women have regular incontinence, compared with men, who report 2 to 7% incidence. The overall prevalence of urinary incontinence in persons 65 years or older living independently in the community is 30% but rises to 50% in institutionalized elderly. The National Institutes of Health report that at least 10 million Americans are incontinent. Incontinence is the most common reason for institutionalizing elderly people. Although incontinence is a major cause of disability and dependence, approximately 70% of cases can be corrected.[18]

Data must be collected to determine the type of incontinence. Four specific types of urinary incontinence are true or total, stress, urgency, and paradoxic or overflow. It must be determined whether the incontinence is acute or chronic. Causes of acute incontinence may include (1) dehydration, which concentrates the urine and can irritate the bladder wall; (2) urinary retention, which may be a side effect of some drugs or a symptom of prostatic enlargement; (3) fecal impaction, which can press on a weakened bladder and obstruct the lower urinary tract; or (4) urinary tract infection, which can irritate the bladder mucosa. Drugs that may contribute to acute urinary incontinence include (1) diuretics, which increase the workload of the bladder; (2) sedatives, which decrease the patient's awareness of the urge to urinate; (3) anticholinergics, which can promote retention and result in overflow incontinence; and (4) antihypertensives, which may relax the smooth muscle of the bladder neck.[53]

The *history* may indicate problems that can contribute to incontinence, such as neurologic or urologic problems. The patient is questioned about the incontinence, such as the number of accidents (urine leakage) daily, type of urine loss (dripping or spurts), and associated activities. During the *physical examination,* the clinician asks the patient to squeeze around his or her finger during the digital rectal examination and the vaginal examination in the woman to check sphincter tone and perineal muscle strength. The genital organs are also examined to determine any abnormalities that may cause incontinence. Urodynamic studies may be performed.[53]

True or Total Incontinence

The patient with true or total incontinence suffers from almost continuous urinary leakage. Some common causes include injury to the urethral sphincter; a vesicovaginal fistula in the female occurring secondary to obstetric, surgical, or radiation injury; or acquired neurologic disease.

Incontinence of urine in an adult male is most often due to bladder outlet obstruction. Three procedures available for *treatment* for the male with true or total incontinence are an artificial sphincter, a silicone-gel prosthesis, and an inflatable prosthesis. These treatments are discussed in Chap. 49.

Fistulas are abnormal openings between two organs or between an organ and the skin that allow passage of secretions and other substances. A urinary tract fistula is suspected when urine leaves the body from an unnatural site, such as the vagina, or when unnatural constituents from the bowel, such as air (called *pneumaturia*) or fecal material (called *fecaluria*), appear in the urine.

A vesicovaginal fistula (Chap. 63) is an opening between the bladder and vagina. True incontinence and uri-

nary tract infection are common findings. A small vesicovaginal fistula is treated by sealing it by coagulation of the epithelium of the fistula tract with an electrode. Larger fistulas are closed surgically, thereby restoring continence. Fistulas that develop following radiation therapy for cancer are more difficult to repair because of the fragile tissues. A permanent urinary diversion may be necessary.

A relatively new procedure for the treatment of true incontinence in men and women consists of collagen injections into suburethral tissue. This is an outpatient procedure done by way of cystoscopy. Studies have shown an 80% success rate for men who were incontinent following prostate surgery and a 96% success rate for women with true incontinence due to intrinsic sphincter deficiency. The procedure is safe, poses fewer risks than major surgery, and is more reasonable in cost.[57]

Stress Incontinence

Stress incontinence refers to the leakage of urine as a result of a sudden increase in intra-abdominal pressure that may occur with sneezing, coughing, or other straining. It occurs more frequently in women with pelvic relaxation resulting from childbirth trauma, loss of tissue tone, and aging.

Conservative Treatment. Conservative treatment of stress incontinence includes consistent Kegel exercises that strengthen the perineal muscles. A *research study* to test the efficacy of bladder training in older women with urinary incontinence (UI) through a protocol of patient education and a mandatory micturition schedule showed the number of UI episodes significantly ($p < .0001$) reduced. The researchers reported that 75% of patients improved by more than 50%.[24] The physician may prescribe drugs that cause contraction of the smooth muscle of the bladder neck, thus enhancing continence. These drugs include phenylpropanolamine (Triaminic) and pseudoephedrine (Sudafed). Estrogen replacements may be prescribed to help maintain vaginal and bladder muscle control in women.

Surgical Treatment. If conservative measures fail, surgical repair is necessary. The bladder neck is elevated by suturing it and the proximal urethra to the periosteum of the superior pubic ramus or the perichondrium of the symphysis pubis. Elevating the base of the bladder and creating a normal ureterovesical angle often restore continence. This surgery is called the *Marshall-Marchetti-Krantz procedure.*

To prevent pelvic infection, an antibiotic is usually administered preoperatively. The patient returns to the urology unit with a Foley or suprapubic catheter in place. The antibiotic is continued, along with a high fluid intake. Very few of these patients can void by the second or third postoperative day, but they ultimately void without residual urine. If a suprapubic catheter is used, it is removed when the patient is able to consistently void about 75% of the total bladder volume.

Nursing Management. Postoperative nursing management includes carefully monitoring the urinary flow from the Foley catheter or the suprapubic catheter. The degree of hematuria should be noted and any signs of hemorrhage reported to the physician immediately. A retropubic drain or drain with suction may be placed during surgery and left in place 2 to 3 days.[84] It should be observed for patency and the characteristics of the drainage should be noted.

The patient may go home with a suprapubic catheter in place and is instructed about how to measure the bladder's residual urine after voiding normally (clamp the suprapubic catheter when able to void, void, then drain the residual urine through the suprapubic catheter after voiding). When the patient is seen at follow-up visits, the physician reviews these volumes and uses them to determine the length of time the suprapubic catheter must stay in place. It may take up to 120 days.

Urgency Incontinence

Urgency incontinence is the involuntary loss of urine that follows a sudden strong desire to urinate. Urodynamic testing is required to truly differentiate the different types of incontinence. Causes of urgency incontinence include bladder disorders such as calculi, diverticula, foreign bodies, and tumors as well as central nervous system disorders such as stroke, dementia, and multiple sclerosis.

The patient should be encouraged to maintain an adequate fluid intake to prevent bacteriuria and increase the functional capacity of the bladder. A bladder "retraining" program (Table 49–4) may be attempted to increase intervals between voiding.[53]

Paradoxical (or Overflow) Incontinence

Paradoxical incontinence is the intermittent loss of urine caused by chronic urinary retention or secondary to a flaccid bladder. Any obstructive bladder disorder, neurogenic bladder, or urinary retention after surgery may result in a large volume of urine in the bladder, leading to overflow incontinence. As additional urine enters the bladder from the kidney, the "overflow urine" produces a sudden desire to void with involuntary leakage of urine if voiding does not occur.

This condition can be the first symptom of benign prostatic hypertrophy in which a man may be retaining up to 500 mL urine.[56] He may feel the need to void every 10, 20, or 30 minutes with some involuntary loss of urine if an appropriate place to void is not immediately available. A very large distended bladder may be palpated.

Catheterization is usually sufficient treatment to relieve retention. The residual volume may be 1 to 3 L. Incontinence resulting from obstruction is treated according to the specific disorder.

General Nursing Management of Patients With Urinary Incontinence

A nursing assessment guide has been developed that can assist in directing nursing management for patients experiencing urinary incontinence.[56] Urinary incontinence is very embarrassing for individuals, causing them to lose their self-esteem and dignity. They may feel they have no control over their bodies, which causes feelings of frustration and hopelessness. The nurse can tell the patient that the feeling of frustration is recognized and that, by working together, perhaps it can be controlled. The patient is encouraged to avoid "giving up" initially and accepting the incontinence as a permanent condition.[77]

A fluid intake of 1.5 to 2 L daily is encouraged and a diet high in fiber is advised.[53] The therapies that are available are explained. The patient is encouraged to void when the urge is felt rather than delaying a trip to the bathroom. Some measures that may be helpful to some patients, depending on the cause of the incontinence, are described.

Increasing Sphincter Tone. Several measures may increase sphincter tone.

- Teach the obese patient the importance of weight reduction so that pressure on the pelvic floor and sphincter is decreased.
- Advise to avoid constipation as straining can also decrease sphincter tone.
- Encourage the patient to exercise the sphincter by starting and stopping the flow of urine three times each time that the bladder is emptied. In addition, encourage to perform the Kegel exercises during the day.
- Encourage the patient on a bladder training program to make a conscious effort to resist micturition for as long as possible and to maintain a sufficient fluid intake.
- Suggest that the use of Velcro fastenings instead of zippers or buttons on clothing that must be removed to void may decrease the delay of voiding.

Protecting the Skin. When all measures have been taken to restore continence and have failed, the patient's skin is protected to prevent chronic irritation and decubitis ulcers. The patient is frequently very depressed at this time. He or she should be encouraged to assist in care, working toward independence when possible. Bladder control may be limited, but the patient may be capable of assisting in cleansing, which can restore some feelings of dignity.

External condom catheters with a leg drainage bag (Fig. 47–13) may be used by men; they can be taught how to make the condom catheters or may use a commercial device. Incontinent pads and diapers may be used by women. The skin should be bathed at least three times a day with soap and water. It is kept as clean and dry as possible.

Evaluation/Desired Outcomes. The patient with urinary incontinence will:

1. Adjust so that a satisfactory lifestyle is achieved
2. Develop a satisfactory method of collecting the incontinent urine
3. Maintain cleanliness of the skin so that breakdown does not occur

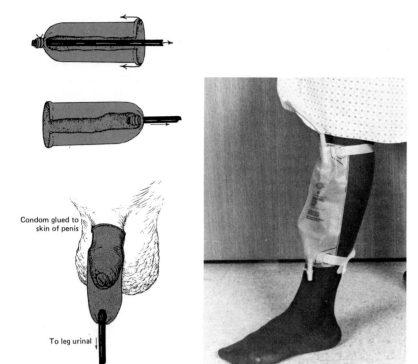

A

Condom glued to skin of penis

To leg urinal

B

Figure 47–13. **A.** Condom catheter that can be devised. After condom of correct size is selected, tip is punctured and attached to drainage tubing with tape or a rubber band. Penis should be clean and dry before condom is rolled onto it. Distal part of condom should be at least 2.5 cm (1 in.) from tip of the penis to allow for erection. Elastoplast is applied to top of condom to anchor it in place. **B.** Leg urinary drainage bag. (**A** *from Smith,*[67] **B** *from Flynn and Hackel.*[26])

■ LEARNING OUTCOMES

After studying this chapter, the nurse will be able to:

1. Discuss the relationships between the anatomic structures of the organs of the urinary system and their functions.

2. Describe the physiologic processes involved in urine formation, including filtration, reabsorption, and secretion.

3. Discuss the renal regulatory mechanisms related to water, electrolytes, acid–base balance, and metabolites.

4. Describe the renal-related functions in regard to renin, erythropoietin, prostaglandins, vitamin D, insulin, and gastrin.

5. Correlate the terms describing the normal anatomy and physiology with the corresponding terms describing the major pathophysiology of the organs of the urinary system.

6. Describe the nursing assessment related to the history of a patient with a problem of the urinary system.

7. Describe the nursing assessment and summarize the key points related to the physical examination of a patient with a problem of the urinary system.

8. Discuss urinary system changes resulting from aging.

9. Describe studies used in diagnosis of disorders of the urinary system.

10. List commonly used nursing diagnoses for patients with problems of the urinary system.

11. Describe the nursing management of patients (a) related to renal insufficiency, (b) needing urethral catheterization, and (c) with urinary incontinence.

REFERENCES

References for Chaps. 47 through 49 can be found on page 1311.

48

Disorders of the Kidneys

Kathy Pike Parker

CHAPTER CONTENTS

Following World War II, nephrology became an important subspecialty in the field of medicine. Prior to this time, the study of renal function and renal disorders focused predominantly on water and electrolyte balance or mechanical problems with urine flow. Later, however, because of the development of many cellular theories and clinically relevant techniques, nephrology became the complex, rapidly expanding field that it is today.[10]

Developments in the field of nephrology have presented the nursing profession with great challenges. Not only is the scientific and theoretical basis of the discipline exceedingly complicated, but the nursing management required by patients with renal disorders continues to grow in complexity with further developments. In addition, renal disorders are associated with multisystemic complications and profound psychosocial ramifications. Thus, the nurse must possess a knowledge base characterized by breadth as well as depth.

■ GLOMERULOPATHIES

The term *glomerulopathies* (also called *glomerulonephropathies*) refers to a group of disorders that are characterized by damage to the glomeruli. Although no classification system for this group of disorders has been universally accepted, they are frequently divided into primary and secondary groups. In *primary glomerular disease,* the glomeruli are the sole or predominant tissue involved. Extrarenal manifestations are the result of the abnormalities that accompany the glomerular injury itself.[10,34] *Secondary glomerular disease* is associated with such disorders as systemic lupus erythematosus, dysproteinemias such as multiple myeloma, infectious and hereditary disorders, and responses to allergens and toxins. Glomerular injury is only a part of an overall process. The glomerulopathies may also be categorized as the nephritic and nephrotic syndromes and as glomerulonephritis.

NEPHRITIC AND NEPHROTIC SYNDROMES OF GLOMERULAR DISEASE

Although there are many different types of glomerular diseases, they seem to manifest themselves either as the nephritic syndrome or the nephrotic syndrome; some glomerular diseases, however, can manifest with features of both.[52,64]

Nephritic Syndrome

This term refers to a group of symptoms that include the abrupt onset of hematuria, mild proteinuria, oliguria, hypertension, and occasionally azotemia.[65]

Pathophysiology. The pathophysiology is related to the underlying cause of the nephritic syndrome, which may include IgA nephropathy, systemic lupus erythematosus, or various types of glomerulonephritis.

Clinical Findings and Diagnostic Studies. In addition to the aforementioned findings, the patient may experience weakness, fatigue, anorexia, and fever. Depending on the etiology, arthralgias, abdominal pain, and a wide variety of other systemic manifestations may be present. Table 48–1 summarizes the major clinical and laboratory findings associated with the nephritic syndrome in comparison to the nephrotic syndrome.

TABLE 48–1

COMPARISON OF CLINICAL AND LABORATORY FINDINGS IN THE NEPHRITIC SYNDROME AND THE NEPHROTIC SYNDROME

Clinical Findings	Nephritic Syndrome	Nephrotic Syndrome
Onset	Usually abrupt	Usually gradual, sometimes acute
Weight gain	May not occur unless renal insufficiency or failure is present	Usually present
Edema	May or may not be present	Usually severe
Blood pressure	Normal to elevated	Usually low (but in rare cases may be elevated)
Protein		
Normal plasma albumin 3.4 to 5 g/dL	Normal	2.5 g/dL but may be less than 1 g/dL
Albumin/globulin ratio 2:1	2:1	1:2
Lipids		
Normal serum triglycerides 30 to 190 mg/dL	Normal	Variable increases
Normal serum phospholipids 125 to 275 mg/dL	Normal	Variable increases
Normal serum cholesterol 140 to 200 mg/dL	Normal	Variable increases
Blood urea nitrogen, normal, 7 to 25 mg/dL	Variable increases	Variable increases
Serum creatinine, normal, 0.5 to 1.5 mg/dL	Variable increases	Variable increases
Urine		
24-Hour urine protein 150 mg/24 hr per 1.73-m body surface area (BSA)	Less than 3.5 g/24 hr per 1.73-m BSA	Greater than 3.5 g/24 hr per 1.73-m BSA; may approach 20 to 30 g/24 hr
Lipiduria (normally none)	Absent	Oval fat bodies and cholesterol esters Free fat droplets Fatty casts
Hematuria (normally none)	Macrohematuria Microhematuria RBC casts Dysmorphic RBCs	May have microhematuria
Pyuria (normally none)	WBCs and granular casts	Usually absent

(Sources: *Brenner and Rector,*[10] *Jacobson and Striker.*[34])

The studies used to diagnose the nephritic syndrome include serum electrolytes, urinalysis, and 24-hour urinary protein determinations. A renal biopsy may also be indicated. Additional studies are listed in Table 48–1.

Treatment. Depending on the etiology and severity of the symptoms, medical treatment for the nephritic syndrome may include various combinations of diuretics, antibiotics, immunosuppressive agents, corticosteroids, plasmapheresis, and/or dialysis.

Complications and Prognosis. Although recovery may be complete, the nephritic syndrome may also be associated with the development of acute renal failure, chronic renal insufficiency, and chronic renal failure. Therefore, systemic complications of acute renal failure, such as congestive heart failure, salt and water retention, hypertension, electrolyte and acid–base disorders, and central nervous system manifestations, may occur.[64] The prognosis of the patient with the nephritic syndrome depends on the cause.

Nephrotic Syndrome

This term, historically referred to as *Bright's disease,* results from an alteration in the glomerular membrane, causing an abnormal loss of protein in the urine (> 3.5 g/24 hr).[52] This results in the clinical findings of hypoalbuminemia, edema, hyperlipidemia, and a hypercoagulable state. Disorders that may cause the nephrotic syndrome include various types of glomerulonephritis, diabetes mellitus, allergies, and primary amyloidosis.

Pathophysiology. *Hypoalbuminemia* is the specific hypoproteinemia most frequently associated with the nephrotic syndrome. Although a correlation does exist between the degree of hypoalbuminemia and the degree of albuminuria, this relationship does not always hold.[34] In addition to renal loss, decreased albumin synthesis by the liver, increased catabolism of albumin, and dietary factors are also important factors. Despite its frequent occurrence, the exact mechanism(s) responsible for the development of hypoalbuminemia in the nephrotic syndrome are not known.

The formation of *edema* is related to the hypoproteinemia in the following ways.

1. The decrease in plasma protein causes a loss of intravascular colloidal pressure, resulting in a shift of fluid from the intravascular compartment to the interstitial space.
2. The shift of fluid out of the intravascular compartment is associated with a reduction in cardiac output and blood pressure (although hypertension may also be seen).
3. Reduction of cardiac output and blood pressure leads to the activation of the renin–angiotensin–aldosterone system, resulting in increased salt and water retention.
4. As the capillaries lose their integrity, the retained fluid leaks from the capillary into the interstitial space, thus increasing edema.

Hyperlipidemia, including an increase in cholesterol, triglycerides, and phospholipids, appears early in the course of the nephrotic syndrome and becomes progressively more severe as the disease progresses. Two major contributing factors are proteinuria and lipiduria, both resulting from the altered glomerular membrane.

The *proteinuria* contributes to a reduction in serum albumin, so the liver is stimulated to synthesize more albumin. This stimulus also appears to trigger the synthesis of lipoproteins. *Lipiduria* may cause a loss of high-density lipoproteins (HDL), resulting in reduced serum levels of HDL. The reduction in HDL is believed to promote elevations in serum cholesterol and triglyceride. As elevated levels of serum cholesterol and decreased levels of HDL are well-established risk factors in the development of cardiovascular disease, patients with the nephrotic syndrome are at a high risk for the development of vascular complications.[34]

The abnormal blood clogging mechanisms producing a *hypercoagulable state* that have been identified in nephrotic patients include the following:

1. A decrease in the activity of factors IX and XII in the coagulation cascade and an increase in fibrinogen activity
2. Abnormalities in the antithrombin and fibrinolytic systems
3. Thrombocytosis (elevated platelet counts)
4. Increased blood viscosity

Clinical Findings and Diagnostic Studies. Table 48–1 summarizes the major clinical and laboratory findings associated with the nephrotic syndrome. The etiology is frequently determined by light, electron, and immunofluorescent microscopy of renal tissue obtained by renal biopsy.

Treatment. Treatment of the nephrotic syndrome depends on the etiology. If a cause is identified, such as an allergen, treatment includes removal of the offending agent. Diuretics, corticosteroids, immunosuppressive agents, and sodium restriction are also frequently used.

If hypoproteinemia becomes severe, salt-poor albumin may be administered intravenously. An expanding body of research supports the notion that a low-protein diet may retard progressive renal damage. It is theorized that lower serum protein levels decrease glomerular filtration pressure and protect the glomerular membranes. A diet low in protein is thus thought to decrease proteinuria, maintain serum proteins, and preserve nephron function.

Complications and Prognosis. The major thrombotic phenomenon that accompanies the nephrotic syndrome is renal vein thrombosis (RVT), indicated by sudden onset of flank pain, costovertebral angle (CVA) tenderness, macroscopic hematuria, and decreasing renal function. Extrarenal thrombosis, including pulmonary embolism, peripheral venous occlusions, and mesenteric, coronary, and femoral occlusions, has also been reported.[34] Anticoagulation therapy, fibrinolytic agents such as streptokinase, and surgical thrombectomy are the treatments. The prognosis of nephrotic syndrome depends on the etiology.

GLOMERULONEPHRITIS

Glomerulonephritis (GN) is a general diagnostic term applied to a number of different diseases that cause inflammation of glomeruli of both kidneys. It is the most common glomerulopathy. Although the varieties of glomerular diseases may cause similar clinical findings, all types have three common factors:

1. The basic problem is an allergic or *immunologic reaction* affecting the glomeruli.
2. The glomeruli are abnormal in some way so that protein leaks through the glomerulus and appears in the urine, producing variable degrees of *proteinuria,* which is a constant sign.
3. Inflammation of the glomeruli leads to microscopic or gross *hematuria.*

Immune complex diseases such as glomerulonephritis begin with the formation of antibodies directed against the invasion of the body by foreign organisms or proteins. Antigens and antibodies then form a protein complex that becomes trapped within the glomerulus and interferes with glomerular function. Acute and chronic glomerulonephritis are discussed next. Table 48–2 describes other types of glomerulonephritis.

Acute Glomerulonephritis

Incidence and Epidemiology. Acute glomerulonephritis (AGN) occurs most commonly after a recent infection of the pharynx, skin, or both with group A beta-hemolytic streptococcus (this condition is also called *poststreptococcal glomerulonephritis* [PSGN]). It may also occur after many other bacterial, viral, and parasitic infections (*infectious glomerulonephritis*), such as pneumococcal or *Klebsiella* pneumonia, staphylococcal sepsis, mumps, malaria, typhoid fever, and hepatitis B.

AGN is principally a disease of children and young adults, but it may occur at any age. The male:female ratio is 2:1.[34]

Nursing Management: Prevention and Reduction of Risk Factors.
Nurses can assist in preventing AGN in the following ways.

1. Encourage prompt treatment of infections in (a) the affected individual, (b) the immediate family, and (c) others who have personal contact with the affected individual to limit the spread of infection.
2. Encourage individuals with a history of AGN to seek medical attention at the onset of any signs of infection: sore throats, skin lesions, or respiratory infections. Additionally, urge these individuals to have a routine yearly examination with appropriate laboratory studies, because glomerular disease can be completely asymptomatic.

3. Emphasize good personal hygiene to prevent the spread of streptococcal infections of the skin.

Pathophysiology. Many features suggest that AGN is an immune complex disease, although the exact nature of the antigen–antibody response in this disease remains unclear.[34] The kidneys become enlarged and pale. The glomeruli swell and narrow the capillary lumen. The damaged glomeruli allow protein and RBCs to leave the bloodstream and enter the urine. These changes are usually reversible.

Clinical Findings. Clinical findings vary from the patient being entirely asymptomatic to having oliguric or anuric acute renal failure. The clinical onset is usually abrupt, with common findings of proteinuria, gross hematuria with a smoky appearance to the urine, and oliguria. Anuria is uncommon. Dysuria may be present in those with severe hematuria.

Clinical findings that are due to the circulatory congestion resulting from sodium and fluid retention occur in slightly more than half the cases. The findings include mild to moderate hypertension with no retinal alterations; edema of face, periorbital area, and hands; dyspnea; cough; positive hepatojugular reflux; ascites; cardiomegaly; gallop heart rhythms; crackles or wheezes; pleural effusion; or even frank pulmonary edema.[34] The patient may hesitate to seek medical attention until fluid congestion is in its advanced stage. Confusion, headache, blurred vision, somnolence, or convulsions may develop. Systemic symptoms such as mild fever, nausea, anorexia, and groin or abdominal pain may also occur.

Diagnostic Studies. Blood chemistry changes related to AGN include (1) increased serum creatinine and BUN levels, (2) decreased hemoglobin of 10 to 11 g and hematocrit of 30 to 34% revealing a mild anemia, and (3) variable increases in serum sodium and potassium.

Creatinine clearance rates may be reduced. Urinalysis will reveal hematuria with RBC casts and proteinuria. Specific gravity will likely be mildly elevated. Urinary sodium is reduced, probably related to the sodium retention because of the depressed glomerular filtration rate (GFR) that frequently occurs in AGN. Throat or skin cultures frequently reveal group A streptococcus, and blood tests often show a positive ASO titer. Serum complement levels are low. A renal biopsy may be indicated for persistence of AGN beyond 2 weeks.[40]

Treatment. The goals for treatment of the patient with AGN are to eliminate the antigen, preserve renal function, prevent cardiac and cerebral complications of hypervolemia, and maintain electrolyte balance. Maintenance of fluid balance is treated with diuretics and control of fluid intake. The degree of sodium and fluid restriction will depend on the general volume status.

Hypertension may be fluid dependent. Thus, antihypertensive drug therapy, including diuretics, may be pre-

TABLE 48–2

TYPES OF GLOMERULONEPHRITIS

Type and Epidemiology	Pathophysiology	Clinical Finding	Treatment and Prognosis
Acute glomerulonephritis	See text		
Rapidly progressive glomerulonephritis (also called *crescentic* or *extracapillary proliferative glomerulonephritis*): most devastating form; disease of adults; tends to occur more in males; can occur in association with infectious diseases or multisystem diseases such as lupus erythematosus	Majority of glomeruli surrounded by large crescentic (sickle-shaped) growths of epithelial cells arising from the lining of Bowman's capsule	Sudden onset following upper respiratory tract infection Nausea, vomiting, and abdominal pain Massive proteinuria Oliguria with hematuria followed by anuria and renal failure in weeks to months Initial hypertension but seldom severe	Dialysis indicated Responds poorly to drug therapy; steroids alone not of great value Anticoagulants may inhibit formation of crescents Treat hypertension *Prognosis:* very poor without initiation of dialysis
Chronic glomerulonephritis	See text		
Minimal change disease: most common form in children; occurs in siblings; occurs in males and females equally	Minimal change in glomerular structures; possibly immunologic process affecting glomerulus, accompanied by good renal function	Viral upper respiratory tract infection common antecedent feature Rapid onset with symptoms of nephrotic syndrome Microscopic hematuria in only 15 to 20% of cases Hypertension uncommon Massive proteinuria	Prednisone, diuretics, cyclophosphamide, or azathioprine (Imuran) Teach family that it is commonly seen in siblings *Prognosis:* favorable; not progressive but may take a remitting and relapsing course
Membranous glomerulonephritis: majority of patients over age 35; males predominate; accounts for 50% of cases of nephrotic syndrome caused by glomerular disease	Thickening glomerular capillary wall, possibly immunologic process affecting glomeruli	Symptoms of nephrotic syndrome with very few or no RBCs in urine Hypertension and azotemia late in disease	*Long-term prognosis* (20-year follow-up): variable—25% have spontaneous remission; 50% have chronic proteinuria or nephrotic syndrome; 25% will progress to end-stage renal disease
Focal glomerulosclerosis: accounts for 10 to 20% of cases of nephrotic syndrome; most cases occur before age 50; seen in heroin abuse and AIDS	Sclerosis of glomeruli; deep glomeruli next to medulla are first to become affected; only some glomeruli diseased initially, but all affected as disease progresses	Distinguishing feature is gross or microscopic hematuria Proteinuria common and sometimes progresses to the nephrotic syndrome Hypertension common	Does not respond well to steroids or to cyclophosphamide *Prognosis:* hypertension and progressive renal failure after variable number of years; recurs in grafted kidneys after transplantation
Membranoproliferative glomerulonephritis (general term with various types): occurs in children and young adults; frequently preceded by upper respiratory tract infection; also associated with various diseases, including infections and neoplasms	Immunologic process; alteration in glomeruli and compression of capillary lumens by immune complexes	Symptoms of nephrotic syndrome Slight or marked hematuria Hypertension early feature and difficult to control	Treat hypertension Responds poorly to drug therapy *Prognosis:* Slowly progressive course to renal failure after 5 to 12 years; recurs in grafted kidney after transplantation
IgA nephropathy (Berger's disease): can occur at any age, but most often in patients over 15 years	Hypercellularity in segments of glomeruli with crescent formation; immunologic process	Hematuria and proteinuria	No treatment has been shown to alter course *Prognosis:* frequently good but slowly progressive disease may develop in up to one half of the patients

(Sources: *Chandrasoma and Taylor,*[14] *Morrison,*[52] *Rose and Rennke.*[64])

scribed. Hyperkalemia is treated by (1) dietary restriction of foods high in potassium; (2) ion exchange resins (Kayexalate, discussed later); (3) dialysis (discussed later), depending on its severity; and (4) limited activity. Whether protein intake is restricted will depend on the degree of *azotemia* (retention of nitrogenous waste products, such as urea) and proteinuria.

Antibiotics are administered initially to prevent further infection that could reactivate the glomerulonephritis. They may be administered for 6 weeks if bacterial endocarditis is present.

Dietary and activity restrictions are discontinued when edema and gross hematuria subside; weight and blood pressure are stable; and the laboratory values of BUN, creatinine, potassium, and sodium return to normal. Forced or prolonged bed rest until the urine is completely normal does not seem to improve or alter the long-term prognosis.[10]

Complications and Prognosis.

Complications include congestive heart failure, renal failure, pulmonary edema, bacterial endocarditis, and hyperkalemia. Hyperkalemia must also be treated immediately because of the associated cardiac arrhythmias. Acute renal failure rarely occurs in the course of AGN.

The course of the illness is usually benign, and treatment with diet and medications is usually sufficient. AGN usually resolves in 6 to 12 weeks, but may take from 1 to 3 years to resolve completely. The mortality rate is usually low. Some patients recover with minimal renal damage, whereas others have irreversible damage that slowly progresses to chronic glomerulonephritis.[34]

Chronic Glomerulonephritis

Chronic glomerulonephritis (CGN) is the clinical expression of a wide variety of glomerular disorders. By definition, the disorder has a protracted course, is often asymptomatic for decades, and is associated with the progressive loss of functional renal mass.[34] In the early stages of CGN, the only manifestations may be minor abnormalities in urinary sediment, increased protein excretion, and mildly reduced renal function. In the final stages, the disorder is characterized by a wide array of biochemical and metabolic disturbances and the uremic state (discussed later).

Incidence and Epidemiology.

The disorder is seen in all ages, but most patients present between the third and fifth decades. Males and females are affected equally.[34] CGN may follow acute glomerulonephritis with persistent microscopic hematuria or proteinuria and may also be associated with other multisystemic diseases.

Nursing Management: Prevention and Reduction of Risk Factors.

Nurses can help to preserve renal function in the patient with CGN in the following ways:

1. Advise the patient to adopt a "healthy-living" plan including good nutrition, weight control, and exercise to assist in blood pressure control.

2. Advise the patient to visit a physician on a regular basis to assess renal function.

3. Emphasize the importance of compliance with diet and medications.

4. Emphasize measures to prevent infections and the importance of notifying the physician should an infection occur.

Pathophysiology.

Renal biopsies are not performed with advanced renal atrophy. The kidneys are almost always significantly reduced in size, and progression of the disease is characterized by a decrease in the thickness of the cortex and a reduced number of functional glomeruli. On microscopic examination, the glomeruli are sclerosed and scarred.

Clinical Findings.

Many patients with CGN have no physical symptoms and discover evidence of renal disease at the time of a routine physical examination. Others will seek medical help after the disorder has progressed to the point that they develop the signs and symptoms of uremia (discussed later). In the early stages of CGN, clinical findings include varying degrees of hypertension and nocturia, which is related to inability of the tubules to concentrate urine. Later, patients may complain of mild headaches, recurrent edema, dyspnea on exertion, orthopnea, weakness, and anorexia.

Diagnostic Studies.

The primary studies include (1) the urinalysis, which reveals proteinuria and hematuria; (2) the KUB and/or renal ultrasound to determine kidney size; and (3) a 24-hour urine for creatinine clearance and protein excretion. As renal function deteriorates, serum chemistries will reveal an increase in BUN, creatinine, potassium, phosphorus (also reported as phosphate), and uric acid levels. Serum CO_2 levels will drop, reflecting the onset of metabolic acidosis. Hematologic studies demonstrate anemia.

Treatment.

Patients having few or no symptoms are seen periodically for routine laboratory studies, physical examination, and blood pressure control. Renal function may be impaired, resulting in proteinuria and hematuria.

Exacerbation of AGN in response to infection in patients with CGN is called *latent chronic glomerulonephritis*.[10] It is characterized by a transient decline in renal function and increased hematuria, proteinuria, hypertension, or edema. It usually resolves spontaneously without any further decline in renal function. No specific therapy exists to arrest or reverse the disease in its progressive form. During exacerbations, the treatment is similar to that for AGN. After progressive nephron loss, dialysis and transplantation are instituted.

Complications and Prognosis.

The ability of the kidneys to regulate the internal environment decreases as additional glomeruli become scarred and functional renal tissue continues to be reduced. Initially, the intact nephrons hypertrophy to compensate, but they eventually become damaged as well and the signs and symptoms of renal insufficiency develop (discussed later). The course of the disorder is usually progressive, and so its outcome is dismal unless dialysis is initiated. CGN is one of the most common causes of chronic renal failure and the need for instituting dialysis.

Nursing Management of Patients With Glomerular Disorders

Nursing management for these patients frequently includes aspects of the care listed in Table 47–7, especially related to fluid balance, hyperkalemia, proteinuria, and infections. Additionally, all aspects of the body's response to immobility should be considered. Aspects of nursing management discussed in Table 47–8 are implemented for patients receiving corticosteroid therapy.

Discharge Planning and Community Care

The patient recovering from a glomerular disorder has the learning needs listed in Table 48–3, which are taught during discharge planning.

During community visits the patients are evaluated for signs suggesting fluid overload and infection. The patient is asked about the frequency of urination, presence or absence of dysuria, and quantity and characteristics of the urine. The blood pressure should be assessed carefully. Detecting elevations of blood pressure at an early stage and instituting

treatment can prevent or delay further renal problems. Nurses may be the first health professionals to recognize the need for further evaluation.

Many years may elapse before signs and symptoms of progressive functional deterioration or renal failure become apparent. Some patients have an acute course followed by progressive functional deterioration. When early signs of complications are recognized or findings are questionable, the patient's physician should be consulted about possible changes in the treatment plan.

Evaluation/Desired Outcomes: Glomerular Disorders. The patient will:

1. Comply with dietary and pharmacologic management
2. Keep scheduled follow-up appointments
3. Develop and maintain a satisfactory lifestyle while incorporating treatment requirements
4. Verbalize and apply appropriate information needed to maintain optimal health and identify complications and seek treatment promptly
5. Be adequately informed and prepared for dialysis and/or transplantation should renal function markedly deteriorate

■ TUBULOINTERSTITIAL NEPHROPATHY

The terms *tubulointerstitial nephropathy* and *tubulointerstitial nephritis* are frequently used interchangeably to describe a group of renal disorders that involve primarily the

TABLE 48–3

TEACHING PLAN: THE PATIENT WITH GLOMERULAR DISORDERS

Teaching Principles	Rationale/Significance
1. Prevent infections: (a) Avoid individuals who are obviously ill. (b) Maintain adequate nutrition. (c) Practice good dental care. (d) Avoid fatigue.	1. Recurrent infections may lead to further glomerular destruction.
2. Seek prompt medical attention for sore throats, skin lesions, or respiratory infections.	2. Initiation of antibiotic therapy by the physician may decrease the severity of the infectious process. In patients with acute glomerulonephritis, it may prevent a recurrence.
3. Report signs that may require immediate medical attention, including (a) blood in the urine or cloudy urine, (b) edema, (c) severe headache, and (d) flank or abdominal pain.	3. These signs may signify activation of glomerular disease.
4. Instruct to seek follow-up care and routine yearly examinations.	4. Glomerular disease can be asymptomatic up to 3 years, but may still be active.
5. Bathe well with soap and water. Avoid dry skin, which will crack and provide an excellent route for infection.	5. Skin infections are associated with acute glomerulonephritis.
6. Take blood pressure as prescribed. Notify the physician of significant elevations.	6. Hypertension can develop as a complication.
7. Consume the prescribed diet.	7. The prescribed protein content may be higher or lower than usual.

renal interstitium and tubules. As tubulointerstitial nephritis implies inflammation—and not all disorders in this classification are inflammatory in nature—the term *tubulointerstitial nephropathy* (TIN) is preferred. This group of disorders is caused by various infections and physical, chemical, immunologic, hereditary, and other forms of injuries to the kidney. Information on specific types of TIN is summarized in Table 48–4.

By a thorough investigation of the patient's clinical and occupational history and laboratory studies, the specific cause of the disorder can frequently be ascertained. Clinically, TIN can be divided into acute and chronic forms. The two most common forms of acute TIN are acute bacterial pyelonephritis, which is discussed in a subsequent section, and acute drug-induced hypersensitivity. The most common cause of chronic TIN is chronic analgesic abuse.

Incidence and Epidemiology

TIN is more frequent in older patients, but may develop at any age. Approximately 20 to 50% of patients with acute TIN develop oliguria or anuria and up to an estimated 30% may eventually require dialysis.[10] The prevalence of chronic TIN in the United States has not been clearly established.[34]

Individuals come into contact with offending chemicals that are used in home, industrial, and agricultural set-

TABLE 48–4

TYPES OF TUBULOINTERSTITIAL NEPHROPATHIES

Type and Pathophysiology	Clinical Findings	Treatment and Prognosis
Acute and chronic tubulointerstitial nephropathies	See text	
Uric acid nephropathy: acute overproduction of uric acid from protein catabolism and increased uric acid production, which causes hyperuricemia, leading to renal failure from tubular obstruction by uric acid crystals in collecting ducts	Increased serum uric acid, uric acid crystalluria, gross or microscopic hematuria, mild proteinuria, increased serum creatinine and BUN Acute onset of oliguria, which can lead to anuria May have symptoms of pyelonephritis as a result of tubular obstruction	Increase urine volume Decrease uric acid formation with xanthine oxidase inhibitor (allopurinol) Increase solubility of uric acid by alkalinizing urine with $NaHCO_3$ to pH greater than 7 *Prognosis:* renal failure usually reversible, but dialysis or transplantation necessary if too advanced
Hypercalcemic nephropathy: results from increased tubular reabsorption of calcium (Hypercalcemia of any cause may lead to hypercalcemic nephropathy. Calcified cellular debris destroys lumen of proximal and distal tubules, which leads to obstruction, atrophy of nephrons, and decreased glomerular filtration rate [GFR]. Once the tubule is lost, the entire nephron is affected. Obstruction by calcium may lead to pyelonephritis.)	Inability to concentrate urine, leading to increased urinary output, polyuria, and nocturia Symptoms of progressive renal insufficiency	Correct hypercalcemia Saline diuresis (0.9% NaCl and furosemide) in those whose urine output is adequate Mithramycin IV to decrease serum calcium (used cautiously as decreased platelet count is a side effect), steroids, and calcitonin Aggressively treat pyelonephritis Low-calcium diet Evaluate parathyroid functioning *Prognosis:* most early functional abnormalities observed can be reversed following correction of hypercalcemia
Hypokalemic nephropathy: potassium depletion over months or years leading to tubular abnormality	Polyuria Excessive thirst GFR maintained Serum potassium less than 3.5	Restore potassium balance Correct underlying cause of potassium depletion (diuretics, GI disturbances—vomiting, diarrhea, laxative abuse) *Prognosis:* once K balance is restored and polyuria disappears, good
Fanconi's syndrome: proximal tubular disorder that results in phosphatemia, aminoaciduria, glucosuria, and losses of bicarbonate, uric acid, potassium, and calcium	Symptoms of osteomalacia or rickets, growth failure, and chronic acidosis Seen in adults with multiple myeloma	Replacement therapy *Prognosis:* variable

(Source: *Brenner and Rector.*[10])

tings. They may be ingested, inhaled, or absorbed by contact with the skin accidentally, intentionally (for suicidal purposes), or from neglect in washing them from the skin. Chronic analgesic use (NSAIDs) can also cause TIN. Substances that frequently cause nephrotoxicity are summarized in Table 48–5. Most cases of acute TIN result from treatment with potentially nephrotoxic drugs. Factors that increase the risk of aminoglycoside nephrotoxicity include high doses and repeated or prolonged courses of treatment, preexisting renal insufficiency, advanced age, dehydration, and cirrhosis of the liver.[34]

The nephrotoxic agents listed in Table 48–5 can produce varying degrees of renal insufficiency or a rapid decrease in renal function. Although acute renal failure frequently occurs, a slow progressive loss of renal function is possible with continued exposure to the offending agent.

Chronic TIN related to analgesic abuse seems to be widespread. Individuals at higher risk are those with chronic conditions associated with pain, such as arthritis or back conditions, who require daily use of these analgesics. Individuals whose work involves contact with antifreeze or insecticides are also more likely to be at a higher risk.

Nursing Management: Prevention and Reduction of Risk Factors

Nurses can assist in preventing toxic nephropathy in the following ways.

1. Identify patients at risk and the presence of associated predisposing factors.

2. Prevent dehydration in patients at risk.

3. Monitor BUN, creatinine, and drug levels in patients receiving aminoglycoside therapy or other nephrotoxic drugs. If a report is reviewed with a significant level (elevated BUN and creatinine or toxic level of drug) that the physician has not had an opportunity to see and the drug is due to be administered, withhold the drug until conferring with the physician.

4. Provide public education regarding the dangers related to use of over-the-counter analgesic medications and improper use of chemicals and poisons.

5. Provide public education for those at high risk. Industrial and public health nursing occupational goals include prevention of injury to individuals. Develop formal and informal inservice educational programs. Remember that some people using these chemicals are unable to read; they may benefit from a slide and audiotape presentation.

Pathophysiology

The kidney is particularly vulnerable to toxic substances because of its rich blood supply and its functions of concentration and secretion. Blood circulates through the kidneys 12 times per hour, so the kidneys are repeatedly exposed to substances in the blood. The kidneys are the site for concentration and secretion of substances, including toxins. Therefore, the tubules are intimately exposed to the toxins.[76]

Clinical Findings

Clinical findings frequently associated with acute TIN include fever, hematuria, and eosinophilia. Severe TIN can produce acute renal failure (discussed in the next section) with clinical findings of anuria, acidosis, fluid overload, and hypertension (unless shock is present). Infection may complicate the condition.

In diffuse or acute interstitial disease, there may be significant clinical findings similar to those associated with the glomerulopathies.[34] Many patients also have nonspecific clinical manifestations of renal insufficiency. By a thorough investigation of the patient's clinical and occupational history and laboratory studies, the specific cause of the disorder can frequently be ascertained.

Clinical findings associated with chronic TIN include nocturia and renal colic from papillary necrosis associated with gross hematuria. Bacterial pyelonephritis also occurs frequently.

Diagnostic Studies

Blood and urine laboratory tests include 24-hour urine, protein, and creatinine clearance studies. Hematuria, sterile pyuria, and mild to moderate proteinuria are usually present.[34] Blood analysis may indicate acute renal failure with azotemia (elevated BUN and creatinine) and hyperkalemia. A decreased carbon dioxide level indicates acidosis. Hemoglobin and hematocrit levels may indicate anemia. Once the

TABLE 48–5

NEPHROTOXIC AGENTS

Analgesics	Nonsteroidal antiinflammatory drugs (NSAIDs), including aspirin
Anesthetic agents	Methoxyflurane, enflurane
Antibiotics	Aminoglycosides, cephalosporins, penicillins, sulfonamides, tetracyclines
Antifreeze	(Ethylene glycol)
Antiulcer regimens	Cimetidine, excess milk and alkali
Chemotherapeutic and immunosuppressive agents	Cisplatin, cyclosporine, methotrexate, mitomycin, nitrosoureas
Contrast media	Iodinated agents
Diuretics	Furosemide, thiazides
Heavy metals	Mercury, arsenic, lead
Organic solvents	Gasoline, kerosene
Pigment nephropathy	Hemoglobin, myoglobin
Poisons	Fungicides, insecticides (chlordane), herbicides (paraquat)
Recreational drugs	Amphetamines, heroin

(Sources: *Brenner and Rector,*[10] *Jacobson and Striker.*[34])

diagnosis of TIN has been made, radiologic testing requiring contrast medium may be temporarily contraindicated to minimize further damage.

Treatment

Treatment includes preventing further exposure to the toxic substance. Large doses of nephrotoxic agents taken intentionally (as in a suicide attempt) or accidentally may be removed with emetics, gastric lavage, peritoneal dialysis, or hemodialysis. Dimercaprol (BAL) may facilitate the removal of heavy metal ions. *Hemoperfusion* (form of dialysis to remove toxic agents from the body by the use of a chemical binder) may be initiated to speed the substance's removal. Some nephron loss will occur, but a slow return to normal renal function is expected after recovery. If acute renal failure (ARF; discussed later) has occurred, management is similar to that for other patients with ARF. Dialysis (discussed later) can maintain the patient's life until the tubular tissue regenerates.

Complications and Prognosis

Acute complications of TIN may include hyperkalemia, volume overload or dehydration, and acid–base disturbances. From 20 to 50% of patients with TIN develop oliguria or anuria, and an estimated 30% may eventually require dialysis.[10] If ARF develops and volume overload is severe, congestive heart failure and pulmonary edema may occur. Complications of chronic TIN include slow progressive loss of renal function. In patients receiving aminoglycoside antibiotics, renal function usually returns to pretreatment levels once the drug has been discontinued.

The prognosis for patients with acute TIN is usually good and renal function frequently returns to normal. The prognosis for patients with chronic TIN is less optimistic and severe renal insufficiency or failure develops, requiring dialysis.

Nursing Management

General supportive care includes prevention of fluid and electrolyte imbalance and acid–base imbalance. Hypertension is controlled with prescribed medications and diet therapy. Infections are treated with antibiotics that are not nephrotoxic. The patient is provided with appropriate food and fluid intake. Nursing management of the patient with acute renal failure is discussed in the next section.

Discharge Planning and Community Care

The following points should be considered in discharge planning and during community visits.

1. If the patient has been exposed to chemicals in the home or work environment that have caused toxicity, help him or her to discover ways of preventing the exposure. A change in occupation may be necessary. Encourage adher-

ing to precautions recommended in the workplace, such as use of gloves and/or masks.

2. When taking the patient's initial history, analgesic overuse may have been discovered. Ask the reason for taking the drug and other ways that have been used of dealing with the pain the patient is experiencing, or discuss ways to deal with the habit that has developed. Assist the patient to deal with the chronic pain (Chap. 10).

3. If the patient appears to be under excess stress and is having difficulty coping with it, explore possible ways of learning to deal with it (Chap. 5).

4. If the ingestion of the toxic agent was an attempt at suicide, urge the patient to seek and/or continue with counseling.

■ RENAL FAILURE

Renal function is not an all-or-none phenomenon. Instead, it exists on a continuum. *Normal renal function* is at one end of the continuum. *Renal impairment* is a state in which the patient is asymptomatic and the small but significant decrease in renal function can be detected only by specific concentration and dilution tests. In *renal insufficiency,* the loss of renal function is great enough to produce symptoms, because the kidneys are unable to meet the demands of dietary or metabolic stress. *Renal failure* is a condition in which the kidneys are unable to meet the normal demands of the body.[59] At the other end of the continuum is *end-stage renal failure* (ESRD); the kidneys are nonfunctional so that dialysis and transplantation are required to sustain life. Table 48–6 lists the changes in clinical findings and alterations in laboratory values along the continuum.

Renal failure is broadly classified as acute and chronic. In acute renal failure, renal function deteriorates rapidly, whereas chronic renal failure develops slowly, sometimes over a period of years or decades. In both situations, renal failure triggers multisystemic abnormalities that predispose the patient to several serious problems requiring complex nursing care.

ACUTE RENAL FAILURE

Acute renal failure (ARF) refers to the rapid deterioration of renal function resulting in accumulation of nitrogenous wastes in the blood (called *uremia* or *azotemia*) and the sudden inability of the kidney to regulate water and electrolyte balance. The wastes include urea and creatinine.[10] ARF develops over a period of hours, days, or weeks. It is usually a reversible process, often self-resolving, but may lead to irreversible renal failure.

ARF may also occur superimposed on chronic renal insufficiency. This form of renal failure is an acute deterioration of function in a patient with preexisting chronic renal abnormalities and is also often reversible within the limits set by the underlying disease.[40]

ARF is diagnosed by obtaining information from the patient's history and laboratory findings. The demonstra-

TABLE 48–6

CONTINUUM OF RENAL FUNCTION FROM NORMAL TO END-STAGE RENAL FAILURE

Stages	Clinical Findings	Alterations
Normal		GFR: 125 mL/min
Renal impairment: normal functioning unless patient is exposed to unusual stress	Asymptomatic	GFR: 50 mL/min Serum creatinine: less than 2 BUN: high normal
Renal insufficiency: easily precipitated by unusual dietary or metabolic stress	Early symptoms of nocturia, polyuria, nausea, weakness, fatigability, anorexia, weight loss	GFR: 15 to 40 mL/min Mild anemia Mild azotemia
Renal failure: normal demands of body cannot be met; may be *acute* or *chronic*	Later, urinary output decreases; volume retention and hypertension	GFR: less than 15 mL/min Serum creatinine: more than 5 mg/dL Azotemia and acidosis Anemia Electrolyte imbalance: hyperkalemia, hypocalcemia, hyperphosphatemia
End-stage renal disease: nonfunctioning kidneys; dialysis or transplantation required to sustain life	Impairment in body systems, manifestations of the uremic syndrome	GFR: less than 5 mL/min Creatinine and BUN: increased markedly Electrolyte imbalances Acidosis

(Source: *Morrison,*[52] *Price,*[59] *Tanagho and McAninch.*[79])

tion of normal-size kidneys on x-ray or renal ultrasound is an extremely important clinical finding that supports the diagnosis of ARF. The finding of small kidneys supports the diagnosis of chronic renal failure.

There are three basic types of acute renal failure: prerenal azotemia, postrenal azotemia, and acute (intrinsic/intra) renal failure (Fig. 48–1). The terminology can be confusing. Prerenal and postrenal azotemia can both lead to acute intrarenal failure. Therefore, acute intrarenal failure is commonly referred to as acute renal failure (ARF).

Prerenal Azotemia

Prerenal azotemia may be defined as a decrease in the glomerular filtration rate (GFR) resulting from renal hypoperfusion. It can be immediately reversed on restoration of renal blood flow and is not associated with structural renal damage.[1]

Epidemiology. Prerenal azotemia in hospitalized patients most commonly results from a combination of hypotension, hypovolemia, and diminished renal perfusion.[34] Some causes of prerenal azotemia are summarized in Table 48–7.

Pathophysiology. Because the kidneys receive 25% of the cardiac output, they are very sensitive to changes in this blood supply. When the renal blood flow is diminished, oxygen and nutrients that support renal cellular metabolism

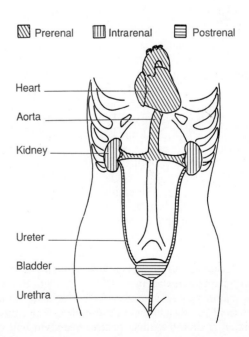

Figure 48–1. Categories of acute renal failure: prerenal, intrarenal, and postrenal.

TABLE 48-7

CAUSES OF PRERENAL AZOTEMIA

Intravascular volume depletion
- Skin losses (sweating or burns)
- Gastrointestinal losses (vomiting or diarrhea)
- Urinary losses (diuretics)
- Hemorrhage

Decreased cardiac output
- Myocardial infarction
- Cardiac failure
- Cardiac arrhythmias
- Cardiac tamponade

Vascular failure caused by vasodilation from such causes as:
- Sepsis (endotoxins produced by gram-negative microorganisms produce vasodilation)
- Anaphylaxis
- Extreme acidosis

Renovascular obstruction
- Renal artery thrombosis
- Renal vein thrombosis

and glomerular filtration are also diminished. Thus, although the kidneys are structurally normal, they become unable to function properly.

Clinical Findings. In prerenal azotemia, one of the earliest changes noted is an increase in tubular reabsorption of sodium and water, reflected in a concentrated urine with a low sodium content. The resulting decrease in urine flow also produces a drop in urea clearance and an elevation in serum BUN without a proportional increase in serum creatinine. The normal BUN:creatinine ratio is 10:1 to 15:1. In prerenal failure it is greater than 15:1. If the perfusion abnormality is not corrected, intrarenal failure may develop. The diagnosis of prerenal azotemia is supported and distinguished from other types of acute renal failure on the basis of urine and blood tests in addition to history and clinical findings.

A *therapeutic fluid challenge* is given (usually 250 mL 5% dextrose in water over a 30-minute period) to ascertain whether the acute renal abnormality is from prerenal or intrarenal causes. The response may be increased by also administering mannitol or furosemide. An increase in the urinary output indicates that the cause is prerenal and additional fluid is needed; no change in the output indicates an intrarenal cause.[42]

Treatment. Treatment of the decreased circulating blood volume is adequate replacement of the needed fluids—blood, plasma, or water—and needed electrolytes or mobilization of fluid in other body compartments. If decreased cardiac output is due to cardiac failure, treatment will depend on the cause. For instance, if the patient had a myocardial infarction and developed heart failure, the treatment

would be to improve the function of the heart as a pump and therefore improve blood flow to the kidneys. The treatment of vascular failure depends on the precipitating cause.

Postrenal Azotemia

Postrenal azotemia is caused by obstruction to the flow of urine. The obstruction may affect one or both ureters, the outlet of the bladder, or the urethra. If bilateral ureteral obstruction occurs, the patient is completely anuric. The causes of obstruction may include (1) calculi, (2) neoplasms of the ureters, bladder, urethra, or pelvic organs, (3) enlarged prostate gland causing urethral obstruction, (4) surgical accidents (inadvertent clamping of the ureters during pelvic surgery) that cause obstruction, and (5) bilateral ureteral instrumentation. Treatment is relief of the obstruction. Prolonged obstruction will lead to intrarenal failure.

Postobstructive Diuresis. After the obstruction has been relieved, renal function can sometimes be significantly altered so that large amounts of solutes and water are excreted. This diuresis is referred to as postobstructive diuresis. Three factors are thought to contribute to its development. *First,* fluid taken orally or administered intravenously before removal of the obstruction can cause volume expansion, which is later excreted. *Second,* solutes such as urea and electrolytes, which were also retained, can act as osmotic diuretics and facilitate the diuresis. *Third,* tubular damage may have occurred during the obstructive phase that inhibits the normal concentrating abilities of the kidney.[10]

The polyuria is usually associated with the excretion of large amounts of sodium, potassium, magnesium, and other electrolytes. Although the condition is self-limiting, the fluid and electrolyte loss that occurs can be life-threatening.

Acute Intrarenal Failure

Acute intrarenal (also called intrinsic renal) failure (ARF) may be defined as a decrease in GFR, usually resulting from renal diseases, renal hypoperfusion, or a nephrotoxin. The GFR is not immediately reversed on termination of the insult; tubular cell damage also occurs. Damage to the tubules secondary to ischemia or toxins is called *acute tubular necrosis* (ATN). The most common type of ARF is ATN.[34]

Incidence and Epidemiology. ATN is induced primarily by the following factors: ischemia, nephrotoxic agents, inflammatory processes, hypersensitivity reactions, intravascular hemolysis (transfusion reactions), systemic and vascular disorders, and pregnancy-related disorders. Acute renal failure occurs most frequently in acute care facilities, reaching an overall incidence of 2 to 5% of hospitalized patients.[1,37] The incidence increases to 10 to 20% in the critically ill.[60]

Nursing Management: Prevention and Reduction of Risk Factors. Because ATN usually occurs in a predictable clinical setting, *anticipation* is the key to prevention. The majority of cases of ATN are caused by shock, blood volume depletion, or toxic substances. Thus, the best way to prevent ATN is to prevent these conditions. The most important nursing interventions that should be implemented for patients at risk include careful monitoring, maintaining adequate hydration, and patient education. Nurses can be exceedingly helpful in preventing ATN in the following ways.

1. In surgical, burned, or traumatized patients or patients in shock, promptly administer prescribed blood and fluids.

2. Administer intravenous fluids, mannitol, and furosemide promptly when they are prescribed for a patient after a muscle-crushing injury, mismatched transfusion, or hemolysis. These therapies may prevent oliguria.

3. Note any significant changes in a patient's urinary output, level of consciousness, temperature, blood pressure, pulse, respiration, or urinary specific gravity that may indicate any of the types of shock and report them to the physician. If hemodynamic monitoring is being done, report changes to the physician.

4. Monitor the patient's overall fluid balance, paying particular attention to the total intake and output over 24-hour periods and changes in weight.

5. Carefully monitor the patient for adequate vascular perfusion periodically. Assess the temperature of the hands and feet and capillary filling, check the blood pressure for orthostatic changes, and monitor filling of the neck veins.

6. Closely observe the patient during administration of a blood transfusion; mismatched blood may cause ATN.

7. Closely monitor patients who are receiving potentially nephrotoxic drugs for sudden changes in urine output and signs of changes in renal function. In addition, monitor the values of the peaks and troughs of the drugs (Fig. 7–4) and report toxic values to the physician immediately.

Pathophysiology. The two most common causes of ATN are renal ischemia and nephrotoxins.

Although *renal ischemia* is the most common cause of ATN, individual patients exhibit varying degrees of sensitivity to a decrease in renal perfusion. In some patients, ATN occurs after a few minutes of hypotension. Others tolerate renal ischemia for hours without showing signs of structural damage to the kidneys. Patients are usually at high risk for developing ATN if the mean arterial blood pressure is less than 70 mm Hg. The most important physiologic changes that result from decreased renal blood flow and that lead to development of ATN are vasoconstriction and decreased glomerular filtration rate. Tubular dysfunction may also develop.[34] In ATN caused by *nephrotoxins,* the initiating mechanism is injury to the tubule cell. The changes that follow are basically the same as those in ischemia.

Renal failure is maintained by (1) persistent renal vasoconstriction, (2) tubular obstruction, (3) leakage of filtrate across damaged tubular epitheluim, or (4) a decrease in glomerular capillary permeability.[34] Tubular compression by interstitial edema and occlusion of the lumen of the tubules by casts and debris leads to necrosis and degeneration of tubular epithelium, which causes oliguria. Altered glomerular permeability, vasoconstriction, and tubular necrosis may allow backflow (or reabsorption) of glomerular filtrate. Total

renal blood flow is reduced by about 50% in patients with ATN. The cause of this reduction is not known. Pathophysiologic changes are summarized in Table 48–8.

Clinical Findings. The most common presenting sign of ARF is sudden oliguria (or occasionally anuria). This is different from the progressive loss of nephrons and slow decline in function seen in CRF. The clinical findings are also different because the body has not had time to adapt to the biochemical changes of uremia, and the patient appears more acutely ill.

ARF proceeds through several well-defined stages: onset, oliguric–anuric stage, diuretic stage, and convalescent stage.

Onset. ARF begins with the precipitating event, which may occur hours or days before the onset of oliguria or anuria. The onset is usually abrupt and associated with ischemia or nephrotoxins.

Oliguric–Anuric Stage. This stage begins when the urine output drops to less than 500 mL per 24 hours. Because the kidney has lost most or all of its regulatory and excretory functions, the patient can experience any of the clinical findings of acute uremia. Acute uremic symptoms may appear within 72 hours. These findings are summarized according to the body systems in Table 48–8.

Although the oliguric–anuric stage usually lasts from 7 to 14 days, it can persist for weeks, depending on the extent of the renal injury. Renal impairment persists throughout this stage, although the healing of renal tissue usually begins within 24 to 48 hours of the insult.

Occasionally, the patient will maintain a normal or above-normal urinary output in the presence of an elevated BUN and creatinine when tubular damage occurs and concentrating ability is decreased. This type of renal failure is known as *nonoliguric acute renal failure.* Patients may still develop the signs and symptoms of acute uremia, but are less likely to retain excess fluid.

Diuretic Stage. The diuretic stage begins when the daily urinary output is greater than 500 mL per 24 hours. The BUN suddenly stops rising, later stabilizes, and finally begins to fall. Although renal healing is also occurring during this stage, the tubule system is frequently unable to satisfactorily concentrate urine. Thus, patients may excrete volumes of urine in excess of 10 L a day and lose substantial amounts of important electrolytes.

Convalescent Stage. The convalescent stage begins when the BUN is stable and lasts until the patient is able to return to normal activity. Complete recovery may require several months. Renal function may never return to baseline, and patients may have significant renal impairment.

Diagnostic Studies. During the *oliguric stage,* blood chemistries reveal elevations of serum creatinine, BUN, potassium, phosphorus, and magnesium, with decreased

TABLE 48-8

ACUTE RENAL FAILURE (UREMIA): PATHOPHYSIOLOGY AND RELATED CLINICAL FINDINGS

Body System	Pathophysiology	Clinical Findings
Fluid and electrolyte status	Kidneys have decreased ability or are unable to regulate fluid and electrolyte balance.	Fluid retention, hypertension, edema, hyperkalemia, hypocalcemia, hyperphosphatemia, hypermagnesemia
General metabolic status	Kidneys have decreased ability or are unable to excrete metabolic wastes.	Increased BUN and creatinine, metabolic acidosis
Urinary system	Kidney damage is reflected in decreased output and presence of abnormal sediment in urine that is produced. Foley catheters are frequently in place to facilitate urine output and measurement; therefore, the risk of infection is high.	Oliguria or anuria; urine sediment—red and white cells, casts, proteinuria; potential for urinary tract infection
Gastrointestinal system	Uremic wastes are retained and exert effects on mucous membranes along GI tract.	Anorexia, nausea and vomiting, stomatitis, constipation/diarrhea, GI bleeding, abdominal distention
Cardiovascular system	Fluid is retained, electrolyte abnormalities (particularly hyperkalemia) are present, and uremia affects pericardial membranes.	Hypertension or hypotension, congestive heart failure, pericarditis, arrhythmias, pericardial effusion, cardiac tamponade
Respiratory system	Hyperventilation is a compensatory mechanism for metabolic acidosis. Pulmonary edema may develop with volume overload. Decreased lung expansion in patient on bed rest, along with the decreased immunologic response seen in acute renal failure, facilitates development of pneumonia.	Hyperventilation, pulmonary edema, potential for pneumonia, depressed cough reflex, hiccups
Hematologic system	Anemia is related to depressed erythropoietin secretion. Uremia decreases platelet adhesiveness and immunologic responses.	Anemia, potential for bleeding and infections
Neurologic system	Accumulation of metabolic wastes may result in alteration of mental status.	Drowsiness, coma, convulsions, myoclonus, psychosis
Dermatologic system	Skin changes result from accumulation of metabolic wastes, calcium and phosphate imbalances, and platelet abnormalities associated with uremia.	Dryness, pruritus, purpura, potential for infection as a result of cracking of the skin

levels of pH, bicarbonate, calcium, hematocrit, and hemoglobin. Frequent blood analyses of serum creatinine and BUN are performed. Creatinine more clearly reflects kidney function; BUN is subject to wider variations, because any condition that increases urea production or nitrogen breakdown in the tissues will increase the BUN.

Urinary findings include decreased volume, mild to moderate proteinuria, casts, cellular debris, red and white blood cells, and increased or fixed specific gravity. Urine sodium may be greater than 40 mEq/L. During the *diuretic stage,* the BUN and creatinine will slowly decrease. The patient may become hypokalemic and develop metabolic alkalosis.

Treatment. The goals of treatment are to (1) treat the underlying cause of ARF, (2) prevent the progression to irreversible ARF, (3) identify serious complications including hyperkalemia, hypervolemia, pericarditis, pneumonia, and other infections, and (4) promote comfort by symptomatic relief of the symptoms of uremia. The major therapies focus on fluid

and electrolyte balance, dialysis, adequate nutrition, treatment of anemia, and prevention of infection. Indications for dialysis include the life-threatening conditions of hypervolemia, uremia, hyperkalemia, metabolic acidosis, pericarditis, and encephalopathy. The patient with ATN is very ill and is usually placed in a critical care unit for close monitoring.

Complications and Prognosis. The complications are the life-threatening conditions listed earlier. The prognosis varies. The mortality rate is 25% in uncomplicated ATN, but greater than 70% in complicated cases (infection, surgery, trauma, and associated injuries).[10,85] Infection is the most common cause of death in ATN.

Nursing Management. Critical observations and effective actions are essential. During the *oliguric–anuric stage,* which is due to the severe tubular damage, the volume of fluids must be administered carefully to avoid hypervolemia. The treatments and related nursing management during this stage are discussed in Table 48–9.

TABLE 48–9

NURSING MANAGEMENT PLAN: THE PATIENT DURING THE OLIGURIC–ANURIC STAGE OF ACUTE RENAL FAILURE

Potential Nursing Diagnoses/Collaborative Problems
- Fluid volume excess, actual or potential related to diminished renal blood flow, electrolyte imbalance
- Nutrition altered, potential for more than body requirements related to dietary indiscretions
- Coping, ineffective individual, related to situational crisis (acute renal failure [ARF])
- Home maintenance, altered, related to extreme fatigue

Goals/Desired Outcomes
- The patient will recover from acute renal failure and complications will be prevented.

Interventions	Rationale/Significance

1. Monitor the volume status; monitor for hypervolemia and/or hypovolemia.
  • Refer to Table 47–7.
  • Weigh the patient frequently.
  • Meticulously provide prescribed volume replacement (usually based on the previous day's urinary output plus insensible water loss of 500 to 1,000 mL).
  • If the patient is alert, plan the intake with him or her over a 24-hour period. Ask if having part of the fluid frozen is preferred so that it will stay in the mouth longer.
  • Measure liquids very carefully.
  • Take into account any liquid in medications and IV fluids.
	1. Intake has to be very closely monitored because there is little or no urinary output.

2. Monitor the patient for electrolyte imbalances; refer to Table 47–7. The following are particularly common in ARF:
A. Observe for *hyperkalemia* (K [potassium] greater than 5.5):
  a. Monitor for a dull headache, abdominal pain, rapid respirations, weakness, nausea, vomiting, general malaise, and decreased pH of arterial blood.
  b. Monitor the ECG rhythm with particular attention to T-wave formation and ventricular arrhythmias. Report any significant findings to the physician immediately.
  c. Treat hyperkalemia as prescribed. Administer the prescribed ion exchange resin (Kayexalate) orally, rectally, or by both routes. Observe for side effects including anorexia, nausea, vomiting, severe constipation, hypocalcemia, and hypokalemia.
           or
  d. Administer prescribed sodium bicarbonate IV or orally. Monitor for signs of inability to tolerate Na loads such as fluid overload.
           or
  e. Administer prescribed calcium gluconate IV.
           or
  f. Administer the prescribed insulin–glucose infusion and observe for signs of hypoglycemia: nervousness, weakness, shaking, diaphoresis, or loss of consciousness.
  g. Teach the patient and family about the relationship of K to diminished kidney function and the importance of avoiding the consequences of hyperkalemia. Instruct the patient about the presence of K in food and medications. Discuss the importance of following a prescribed diet, avoiding foods high in K.
	2. Electrolyte imbalances are common in acute renal failure.
	
	  a. These symptoms may aid in the diagnosis.
	
	  b. Peaked T waves and ventricular arrhythmias are frequently associated with hyperkalemia. Cardiac arrhythmias are a frequent cause of death in these patients.
	  c. Kayexalate contains sodium, which exchanges with potassium in the GI tract, enhancing removal of potassium.
	
	  d. Sodium bicarbonate forces potassium into the cells. This is a temporary correction.
	
	  e. Calcium gluconate reverses the cardiotoxic effects of hyperkalemia and prevents cardiac arrest temporarily.
	  f. The insulin–glucose infusion forces potassium to shift into the cells. This is a temporary correction.
	
	  g. Including the patient in the treatment of prevention of hyperkalemia is important.

(Continued)

TABLE 48–9   *(Continued)*

NURSING MANAGEMENT PLAN: THE PATIENT DURING THE OLIGURIC–ANURIC STAGE OF ACUTE RENAL FAILURE

Interventions	Rationale/Significance
B. Monitor for *hypokalemia* by observing ECG changes: lengthened QT interval, changes in the deflection of the T waves, and development of a U wave.	B. Hypokalemia may develop as a side effect of treatment.
a. If a patient is receiving digoxin, assess for digitalis toxicity.	a. Digoxin toxicity may be precipitated by hypokalemia and inability to excrete the drug in the urine.
b. Teach the patient and significant others about the relationship of K to cardiac problems.	
C. Observe for *hypocalcemia:* Monitor serum calcium levels, along with serum pH and albumin levels. Assess for signs of hypocalcemia, such as muscle weakness and tetany.	C. Hypocalcemia usually develops because of the kidney's inability to produce 1,25-dihydroxycholecalciferol, which is necessary to convert vitamin D to a form that can assist in absorption of calcium from the GI tract. Serum pH and albumin can alter the clinical effects of hypocalcemia: Acidosis and hypoalbuminemia decrease protein binding of calcium and protect against tetany.
D. Observe for *hyperphosphatemia:* Monitor serum phosphate levels. Administer prescribed phosphate-binding antacids.	D. Hyperphosphatemia may result because of the kidney's inability to excrete phosphate and because of the inverse relationship to calcium levels.
E. Observe for *hypermagnesemia.* Monitor serum magnesium levels. Assess for signs of hypermagnesemia: initially hypotension; later a flapping tremor (asterixis), lethargy and slow speech, and maybe nausea and vomiting. At harmful levels may have loss of deep tendon reflexes, depressed respirations, and coma.	E. Serum magnesium may be slightly elevated because of decreased excretion. It can reach dangerous levels if the patient is taking magnesium-containing laxatives or antacids, or has marked tissue breakdown or severe acidosis.
3. Observe for *metabolic acidosis:* Monitor the serum CO_2 level. Confer with the physician if it is less than 15. Administer prescribed bicarbonate. Observe for related sodium retention. Monitor for hyperventilation, deep respirations, nausea, vomiting, and altered mentation.	3. Metabolic acidosis may develop because of decreased excretion of hydrogen ions and decreased concentration of plasma bicarbonate. Metabolic acidosis stimulates compensatory respiratory alkalosis to eliminate excessive CO_2.
4. Observe for signs and symptoms of acute uremia (Table 48–8).	4. Uremic symptoms can develop within 72 hours of the onset of ARF.
5. Monitor serum BUN and creatinine levels. Note the ratio between the two.	5. See Table 48–8 for related pathophysiology.
6. Monitor the genitourinary system: Note urine output, specific gravity, urine osmolality, urine electrolytes, and urinary sediment. Provide meticulous catheter care and send urine cultures as indicated. Check prescribed medications, noting changes in dosage and administration required in renal failure.	6. Urine output is usually absent or decreased in ARF, although nonoliguric acute renal failure also occurs.
7. Monitor the gastrointestinal system: Observe for anorexia, nausea, vomiting, stomatitis, diarrhea, and constipation. Monitor all vomitus and feces for blood. Provide meticulous mouth care.	7. GI abnormalities occur in acute uremia.
8. Monitor the cardiovascular system. Monitor fluid status. Monitor pulse and blood pressure for abnormalities. Monitor closely for signs and symptoms of pericarditis, pericardial effusion, and tamponade.	8. Cardiovascular complications also occur in acute uremia.
9. Monitor the respiratory system: Perform a chest assessment. Encourage the patient to cough and deep breathe.	9. Infection, particularly pneumonia, is a common cause of death in patients with ARF.
10. Monitor the hematologic system: Monitor the CBC, noting particularly the hematocrit and WBC. Observe the patient for bleeding and infection.	10. The most common cause of death in ARF is infection.
11. Monitor the neurologic system: Monitor for drowsiness, disorientation, coma, delirium, psychosis, or convulsions.	
12. Monitor the dermatologic system: Closely monitor for breaks in the skin integrity. Provide excellent skin care.	

Interventions	Rationale/Significance
13. Provide optimal nutrition. Provide the prescribed diet with a sufficient amount of carbohydrates, calories, and protein. Carefully record the intake.	13. The patient in ARF is usually in a hypercatabolic state. Protein intake should be of high biologic value. To prevent rapid rise of serum BUN, protein may be restricted. Carbohydrates prevent protein from being used for energy.
14. Assist with hemodialysis or peritoneal dialysis. Assess the patient before, during, and after treatment. (See the section on Dialysis.) Adequately prepare the patient and significant others psychologically for treatment.	14. Dialysis may be required to maintain the patient.
15. Provide consistent psychologic support by listening and allowing the patient time to express his or her feelings. Support the patient and family during the acute illness. Provide adequate education to the patient and family.	15. Acute illness, loss of ability to concentrate, and depression may be very anxiety producing for the patient and family.

In the *diuretic stage* or period of tubular regeneration, hypovolemia must be avoided. The nursing management for the patient during this stage includes those interventions listed in Table 48–9 for any continued abnormalities and in Table 47–7 with emphasis on the following parts: hypovolemia, electrolyte disturbances, preservation of renal function, and potential for infection.

After recovering from the acute stage of the illness, the patient will be placed on a medical or extended care unit. If ARF has progressed to severe CRF, dialysis treatments will begin. The vital signs, cardiopulmonary status, fluid balance, and blood and urine studies need to be monitored carefully. Any infection must be promptly treated.

 Discharge Planning and Community Care

During discharge planning, the patient and family will need to know the extent of renal recovery or impairment, diet necessary to maintain optimum health during recovery, any medications to continue, and symptoms of infection. Once the patient has been discharged, follow-up care will be necessary to monitor the blood chemistries and clinical state.

Evaluation/Desired Outcomes: Acute Renal Failure. The patient (or with the family's assistance) will:

1. Be aware of any residual renal damage present and the increased susceptibility to further renal damage
2. Refrain from use of potential nephrotoxic substances
3. Be able to verbalize any dietary restrictions
4. Understand the name, dose, purpose, frequency, and side effects of any prescribed medications
5. Keep scheduled clinic appointments
6. Increase activity as tolerated
7. Achieve a lifestyle compatible with his or her physical condition and incorporate those changes necessary for health and well-being

The Hepatorenal Syndrome

Hepatorenal syndrome is a broad term used to describe a unique form of ARF that develops in patients with progressive liver disease who have little or no history of impaired renal function. Impairment of renal perfusion secondary to intrarenal vasoconstriction is thought to be the primary cause of the renal failure.[64] Renal blood flow is usually one half or less of normal.

This syndrome occurs in patients with cirrhosis, usually with alcoholic liver disease. The clinical findings of portal hypertension (discussed in Chap. 56) are present, and the majority of patients develop hepatic coma. Renal failure frequently starts after a decrease in fluid volume. Oliguria develops progressively and is the hallmark of the syndrome. Significant azotemia develops and progresses slowly.

Treatment may include dialysis. The prognosis is grave.[40] Nearly all these patients die within days to weeks of its onset. Death may result from factors other than or in addition to ARF. Although renal function is impaired, the structural units of the kidney remain normal, and these kidneys have been successfully used as donor organs in kidney transplantation. Combined nursing management related to the liver disorder and also to the therapies to attempt to restore renal function is needed.

CHRONIC RENAL FAILURE AND END-STAGE RENAL DISEASE

Chronic renal failure is defined as a substantial reduction of the glomerular filtration rate that has persisted for years or even decades as a result of permanent kidney damage. Up to 80% of renal function may be lost before the condition is discovered. CRF frequently progresses to terminal or end-stage renal disease (ESRD), which requires therapy with dialysis (treatment to remove toxic wastes, electrolytes, and excess fluid; discussed later) or transplantation to sustain life. Although the conservative management of the patient with CRF is addressed in this chapter, the primary focus is on the care of the patient with ESRD who requires dialysis.

Incidence and Epidemiology

Historically, kidney disease has been a source of much interest and speculation, primarily because of the successful development of chronic, maintenance dialysis and renal transplantation. Yet amid this interest and speculation emerged a controversy over selection of patients. Before 1973, selection of patients for chronic dialysis was based mainly on social class considerations and social worth more often than rehabilitative potential. Some criteria included "age, medical suitability, family environment, criminal record, economic status (income, net worth), willingness to cooperate in the treatment regimen, likelihood of vocational rehabilitation, psychiatric evaluation, marital status, educational background, and occupation."[23] In an attempt to provide equal access to health care, Congress passed legislation (PL92-603) in 1973 that extended Medicare benefits to virtually all ESRD patients. The number of patients receiving treatment increased tremendously, and the cost increased substantially.

Because of the huge cost, information was greatly needed to assess the effectiveness of the ESRD program and the impact on the lives of those involved. Prior to 1986, only two large-scale studies had been conducted (in 1969 and 1978) about the ESRD population. In 1969 information was collected from 93 of 110 centers providing chronic dialysis[35]; the total number of patients in the study was 689, representing 81% of the total dialysis population. The average dialysis patient at that time was white, middle-aged, educated, married, and working.

The study conducted in 1978 reflected the impact of Medicare legislation selection procedures.[11] The population of 70,000 became more equally distributed among the races, sexes, educational and income levels, and became significantly older. In 1990, Medicare costs for about 150,000 ESRD patients were over $5 billion, which was about 84.1% of total program expenditures.

As of December 1991, approximately 220,000 ESRD patients in the United States were receiving dialysis in 2,202 dialysis centers.[82]

Nursing Management: Prevention and Reduction of Risk Factors

Among the leading causes of renal failure are diabetes, hypertension, glomerulonephritis, and cystic kidney diseases.[82] Prevention or delay of renal failure is related to appropriate treatment of these disorders. Appropriate treatment of congenital abnormalities may delay renal failure.

Pathophysiology

As renal tissue is irreversibly lost by parenchymal disease, the intact nephrons hypertrophy. A consequence is inability to concentrate urine adequately. In an attempt to continue excreting the solutes, a large volume of dilute urine is passed. Thus, two early symptoms of CRF are polyuria and nocturia, followed later by oliguria and anuria. As renal function continues to deteriorate, the number of functioning nephrons declines, the kidneys become small and con-

tracted, GFR decreases further, and the body is unable to normally rid itself of water, electrolytes, and waste products.

Clinical Findings

The *uremic syndrome* is a group of clinical findings affecting every system of the body that occurs in patients with CRF. Although the term *uremic* implies that the syndrome occurs in response to elevations in blood urea nitrogen, the syndrome actually describes the body's total response to loss of renal function as listed below. Figure 48–2 depicts the clinical sequelae of chronic renal failure.

Fluid, Electrolyte, and Acid–Base Abnormalities. As renal function declines, the kidneys are unable to maintain fluid, electrolyte, and acid–base balance. Although patients with CRF may sometimes become volume-depleted, fluid retention is more common.

The most common electrolyte abnormalities in patients with CRF include hypernatremia or hyponatremia, depending on the free water load; hyperkalemia; hyperphosphatemia; and hypocalcemia. The rationales for these electrolyte

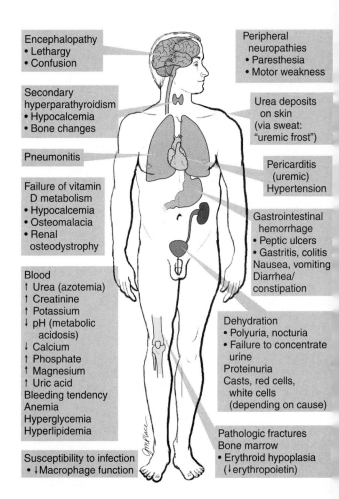

Figure 48–2. Clinical sequelae of chronic renal failure.

abnormalities are discussed in Table 48–9. Hypermagnesemia may also develop, and so it is important that these patients avoid taking magnesium-containing medications, such as antacids. The reasons for the metabolic acidosis and hyperventilation have been discussed previously.

Metabolic Manifestations. The most important metabolic derangements in CRF are carbohydrate intolerance, abnormal protein metabolism, and increased lipids.

These patients frequently have *carbohydrate intolerance* with abnormal handling of glucose. Circulating levels of insulin are higher than normal but are less effective. The peripheral use of insulin is decreased; however, the effectiveness of the insulin is usually sufficient to prevent hyperglycemia. The need for exogenous insulin in the patient with diabetes is usually decreased.

The waste products of *protein metabolism,* such as BUN, accumulate, requiring protein restriction. Adequate intake of essential amino acids is important to prevent severe catabolism. The most common *lipid abnormality* is hypertriglyceridemia, resulting from increased synthesis and impaired removal of the triglycerides.

Neurologic Manifestations. Central, peripheral, and autonomic nervous system problems occur in the uremic syndrome. The *central effects* include headache, lassitude, apathy, drowsiness, and insomnia accompanied by daytime drowsiness. As uremia worsens, changes in memory, somnolence, confusion, and coma can develop but are usually prevented by the institution of dialysis therapy. Seizures occur in severely uremic patients but can also develop in stable patients on chronic dialysis. Behavioral changes include personality changes, increased irritability, emotional lability, depression, and decreased libido. Cranial nerve involvement may result in decreased vision and smell.

Peripheral nervous system effects include paresthesias in the lower extremities, painful dysthesias (abnormal skin sensations), decreases in deep tendon reflexes, gait changes, foot drop, and asterixis. Muscle twitching and myoclonic jerks (the restless leg syndrome) are painful, annoying, and interfere with sleep because they often become worse at night.

Autonomic nervous system abnormalities are probably related to a decreased responsiveness of the baroreceptors. They include failure to develop bradycardia in response to hypertension or tachycardia in response to hypotension.[34] Depression of the cough reflex may also be associated with autonomic nervous system dysfunction.

Cardiovascular Manifestations. The most frequently occurring cardiovascular complication is hypertension, which is usually volume dependent (becoming worse as more fluid is retained). The hypertension may sometimes be related to decreased renal perfusion and activation of the renin–angiotensin system. If not controlled adequately, hypertensive encephalopathy may develop accompanied by headaches, seizures, coma, and strokes. Hypertension also increases the risk of myocardial infarction. Severe fluid retention may lead to development of congestive heart failure. Edema is a very common finding. Cardiac arrhythmias may occur as a result of hyperkalemia, acidosis, or transient myocardial ischemia.

Pericarditis frequently occurs in patients with either ARF or CRF. Atrial fibrillation is a potential complication of pericarditis. Pericardial effusion and cardiac tamponade can also develop.

Evidence exists to support the belief that arteriosclerosis and atherosclerosis are accelerated because of the hyperlipidemia. Left ventricular hypertrophy often develops as a result of the increased workload placed on the heart from hypertension, atherosclerosis, and anemia.

Respiratory Manifestations. Respiratory manifestations include increased susceptibility to infections, pulmonary edema, pneumonitis (uremic lung), and pleuritis with or without pleural effusion. Pneumonia is a frequent cause of death. With infection, the sputum is thick and tenacious. In pulmonary edema, the sputum is thin and frothy. The cough reflex may be depressed. An increase in the respiratory rate may occur as a compensatory response to metabolic acidosis. The odor of ammonia, caused by the breakdown of urea on mucous membrane, may be noted on the breath.

Dermatologic Manifestations. Integumentary problems are particularly uncomfortable for the patient. The eccrine (sweat) glands become smaller and perspiration decreases. Sebaceous gland oil production decreases, which results in dry, scaly skin. Pruritus and a tickling or crawling sensation cause scratching and may lead to skin breakdown. *Uremic frost,* a white powderlike substance seen on the face and trunk, may also form. This condition is rarely seen today as dialysis is usually initiated before it develops. The skin color may be altered to a bronze or tan hue because of the collection of pigments that are normally excreted in the urine. Pallor from anemia is also present. Ecchymosis and purpura secondary to capillary fragility can occur. The nails become thin and brittle and are often pitted or ridged. The dry, brittle hair falls out and breaks easily.

Gastrointestinal Manifestations. Anorexia, nausea, and vomiting are common GI problems that may be related to mucosal alterations from uremia. Although diarrhea may be severe, constipation is also common and is a side effect of the phosphate binders patients take with meals to decrease serum phosphate levels. Patients complain of a metallic or salty taste in the mouth that is probably related to the high concentration of urea in the saliva, which further decreases their appetite. Spontaneous gingival bleeding with frequent episodes of stomatitis occurs. GI bleeding is common and may be related to abnormalities in clotting mechanisms and high circulating levels of gastrin. Although GI bleeding is common in renal failure, there does not appear to be a specific increase in peptic ulcer disease.

Skeletal Manifestations. With loss of renal function, production of 1,25-DHCC, a form of vitamin D, is decreased, causing decreased intestinal absorption of calcium, so hypocalcemia is frequently seen in patients who have CRF. Serum phosphate levels usually increase as a result of its presence in foods and/or tissue breakdown.

In normal circumstances, parathyroid hormone (PTH) is released in response to decreased calcium levels and causes increased tubular reabsorption of calcium, decreased reabsorption of phosphate, and release of calcium ions from bone.[34] In CRF, the renal mechanisms for calcium and phosphate regulation are nonfunctional. To elevate the calcium level, calcium ions are absorbed from the bone into the blood. These abnormalities can lead to the development of secondary hyperparathyroidism and severe bone disease.

Calcium phosphate crystals can deposit in soft tissues so that areas in the joints, myocardium, brain, lungs, skin, blood vessels, and the conjunctiva become calcified. This process, known as *metastatic calcification,* causes further reduction of serum calcium levels. If extensive deposits occur in vital tissues, the process can be lethal.

In *secondary hyperparathyroidism,* the elevated PTH levels continue to "pull" calcium ions out of the bone, leading to further calcium phosphate deposits and worsened hypocalcemia. The results of this vicious cycle in the patient with CRF are probably the most important factors in the development of *renal osteodystrophy* (pathologic changes in bone as a sequela of CRF); it takes several forms. In *osteitis fibrosa,* severely increased bone reabsorption causes a thinning of cortical bone and its replacement by fibrous tissue. Skeletal fractures and deformities with joint pain and dysfunction follow. *Osteomalacia,* or defective mineralization of bone, causes bone pain, tenderness, and skeletal deformities that may be accompanied by muscle weakness and hypotonia. A waddling gait and inability to walk may result. *Osteoporosis* (reduced quantity of bone and/or atrophy of skeletal tissue) may be the most common form of renal osteodystrophy.[10] The major clinical symptoms associated with renal osteodystrophy are fractures, bone pain, and muscle weakness. Muscle weakness is usually reflected in the patient with CRF by difficulty in walking.

Hematologic Manifestations. The anemia of CRF is related to a decreased production of erythropoietin and is usually normochromic and normocytic. Other factors that aggravate the anemia include:

• Shortened RBC lifespan (nearly one half of normal) caused by the abnormal chemical environment resulting from uremia
• Decreased erythropoietin production (the smaller kidneys produce less erythropoietin)
• Bone marrow suppression resulting from the uremic environment
• Vitamin deficiencies (folic acid is a water-soluble vitamin lost during dialysis)
• Iron deficiency because uremic patients have decreased absorption of oral iron from the GI tract and diminished RBC incorporation of iron
• Chronic blood loss associated with hemodialysis or low-grade GI bleeding (patients who have undergone bilateral

nephrectomies usually exhibit a marked anemia and a hematocrit of 16 to 18% because there is no kidney tissue producing erythropoietin)

Fatigue, weakness, dyspnea on exertion, and cold intolerance may accompany the anemia.

WBC counts are usually normal although the cells are less responsive to infection than normal. A qualitative defect in platelet function develops that increases bleeding time.

Reproductive System Manifestations. Patients with ESRD experience a wide variety of problems related to sexual and reproductive functioning. The multifactorial causes include hormonal imbalances, psychologic stress, hypertension, medications used to treat hypertension, anemia, and malnutrition.

Common to both sexes is the loss of libido that frequently becomes worse as the uremia increases. In the male, sperm counts are abnormally low and impotence is a significant problem. Anemia, hypertension, atherosclerotic changes, and low testosterone levels may be contributing factors. In the female, plasma estrogen and progesterone levels are usually low. Increased prolactin levels may contribute to the high incidence of amenorrhea and infertility seen in this group.

Symptoms Most Bothersome to Patients. According to the data collected in the National Kidney Dialysis and Kidney Transplantation Study, the symptoms reported by over one half of all ESRD patients as being most bothersome overall include (1) tiring easily or no energy, (2) weakness or lack of strength, and (3) difficulty sleeping. Other commonly reported symptoms included aches, swelling, sick feeling, cramping pain, anxiety, and headaches.[32]

Diagnostic Studies

Table 48–10 lists the changes that occur in laboratory studies related to such severely decreased renal function in CRF that dialysis must be instituted.

Treatment

The goals of conservative treatment of the patient with CRF are to (1) preserve renal function, (2) postpone or eliminate the need for definitive treatment (dialysis and transplantation), (3) improve body chemistries, (4) reverse organ system alterations when possible, and (5) provide comfort and an improved quality of life. These goals are reached by monitoring the level of renal function periodically, and by the patient's taking the appropriate prescribed medications and consuming a diet based on monitored laboratory and clinical findings.

The extent to which the kidney function is preserved must be determined. Renal function may be preserved by relieving obstructions, treating infections, removing nephrotoxic agents, and controlling hypertension and diabetes when present. If the patient follows dietary restrictions and takes the prescribed drugs, the workload of the

TABLE 48–10

LABORATORY VALUES IN UREMIC PATIENTS ON DIALYSIS AND RELATIONSHIP TO DRUG THERAPY

Laboratory Study Normal Value	Typical Value in Dialysis Patient	Indicates Potential Danger to Patient	Drug Therapy and Pertinent Information
Blood urea nitrogen (BUN) 8 to 25 mg/dL	60 to 90 mg/dL	>100 mg/dL	There is no drug therapy to lower this uremic toxin. Diet and dialysis are the only methods of control.
Creatinine 0.6 to 1.2 mg/dL	10 to 15 mg/dL in 70-kg person	>15 mg/dL in 70-kg person	There is no drug therapy to lower this uremic toxin. Dialysis is the only method of control; it is not diet dependent.
Potassium (K) 3.5 to 5.0 mEq/L	3.5 to 5.0 mEq/L	>5.5 mEq/L <3.0 mEq/L	*Kayexalate* can be mixed with ginger ale to make it more palatable. *Potassium supplement* (use with caution)
Carbon dioxide (CO_2) 22 to 30 mEq/L	18 to 21 mEq/L	<15 mEq/L	*Sodium bicarbonate* *Shoals solution*
Sodium (Na) 135 to 145 mEq/L	135 to 145 mEq/L	>150 mEq/L <120 mEq/L	When the patient is on $NaHCO_3$ and Kayexalate (a Na-containing resin), watch for hypernatremia. Restrict free water intake.
Calcium (Ca) 9 to 11 mg/dL	9.0 mg/dL	<8.0 mg/dL >11 mg/dL	*Calcium* (Titralac, calcium carbonate) *Vitamin D* (calcitriol, Rocaltrol [oral], Calcijex [IV]) Calcium supplements and Rocaltrol are usually withheld.
Phosphate (PO_4) 2.5 to 4.5 mg/dL	2.5 to 4.5 mg/dL	>5.0 mg/dL	*Phosphate binder* (Amphojel, Basaljel, Alternaljel) If Ca × PO_4 is greater than 70 mg/dL, calcium and/or vitamin D will be discontinued to prevent tissue calcification when these two elements precipitate. PO_4 binders will be emphasized. When Ca is slightly low and PO_4 is not at dangerous levels, vitamin D will be given first to use Ca available in intestine. If Ca is very low and PO_4 is not at dangerous levels, both Ca and vitamin D may be prescribed.
Magnesium (Mg) 1.5 to 2.5 mEq/L	Normal	7 mEq/L	Ask if the patient is taking Mg-containing antacids or laxatives. They should be avoided.
Albumin 3.5 to 5.0 g/dL	3.5 to 5.0 g/dL	<3.5 g/dL	There is no drug therapy for low albumin and total protein. A diet of high biologic protein, including eggs, will be emphasized if the patient is on dialysis. Salt-poor albumin IV may be used in acute situations.
Total protein 6.0 to 8.0 g/dL	6.0 to 8.0 g/dL	<5.0 g/dL	
Hemoglobin (Hgb) 12 to 18 g/dL	7 g or more (nephric patient) 4 to 5 g (anephric patient)	Danger range varies greatly; considered dangerous when patient becomes symptomatic	*Folic acid* is dialyzable and must be replaced. Teach patient to take after dialysis. *Recombinant erythropoietin* is being used successfully in this population.
Hematocrit (Hct) 36 to 46%	20 to 25% (nephric) 16 to 18% (anephric)	Danger range same as above	Hypervolemia and hypovolemia can produce false low and high values, respectively.
Iron saturation 20 to 50%	> 20%	<20%	Iron dextran (*Imferon*) IV and/or *ferrous sulfate* PO. Do not administer more than 100 mg Imferon at one time. Give slowly IV over 5 minutes. Watch closely for anaphylactic reaction. Oral iron is not absorbed well in uremic patients but is used when patient is allergic to Imferon. Do not administer with phosphate-binding agents. Iron and RBC values must be monitored monthly when iron supplements are prescribed. When iron is administered IV, hemosiderosis may develop (deposits of iron in liver, lungs, adrenals, skin) because the iron is injected directly into the bloodstream. When a drug is given orally, the amount the body needs is absorbed into the blood.

(Continued)

TABLE 48–10   *(Continued)*

LABORATORY VALUES IN UREMIC PATIENTS ON DIALYSIS AND RELATIONSHIP TO DRUG THERAPY

Laboratory Study Normal Value	Typical Value in Dialysis Patient	Indicates Potential Danger to Patient	Drug Therapy and Pertinent Information
Uric acid 2.8 to 7.8 mg/dL	<10 mg/dL	>10 mg/dL	*Allopurinol* in reduced dosages if symptomatic of gout
Glucose 70 to 110 mg/dL	65 to 120 mg/dL 200 mg/dL for diabetic	Variable high	Insulin is partially excreted by the kidneys; its half-life is increased when the kidneys have failed. The patient may require a lower dose.
Hepatitis B surface antigen	Negative	Positive	Screening of dialysis patients for hepatitis B must be done monthly. Vaccination against hepatitis B is now available— Hepatovax.
Bilirubin total 0.1 to 1.2 mg/dL	0.1 to 1.2 mg/dL	Variable increases; *rate* of increase more significant than actual result	If elevated, suspect hepatitis.
Cholesterol 180 to 200 mg/dL	180 to 300 mg/dL	Variable increases	Monitor these values for significant increases; possibly decrease foods high in saturated fats.
Triglycerides 10 to 190 mg/dL	10 to 190 mg/dL	Variable increases	

(Sources: *For normal values, Kee*[36]; *for cholesterol values, Corbett.*[17])

kidneys will be decreased, volume balance will be maintained, body chemistries will be improved, and the patient's well-being will be increased. The patient's and family's understanding and cooperation will be vital to the success of the prescribed therapeutic program.

When to Begin Further Treatment. These patients will no longer be able to follow conservative treatment when (1) the creatinine clearance falls significantly (usually < 5 to 10 mL/min), (2) GRF decreases to approximately 5 mL/min or less, (3) serum creatinine rises to 6 mg/dL, (4) general uremic symptoms develop, (5) pericarditis or congestive heart failure persists, (6) peripheral neuropathy or renal osteodystrophy progresses, and (7) severe mental dysfunctions or psychosis develops.

To maintain an acceptable blood level of uremic toxins, dialysis or a renal transplant is necessary. Dialysis requires the patients to make changes in their lifestyles to provide time for the treatments. Options in therapy should be discussed with the patients and their families. This gives them time to prepare for the commitment necessary for the management of end-stage of renal failure and to consider in advance the changes in occupation, residence, and finances.

Pharmacologic Management. Table 48–10 lists pertinent information regarding drug therapy. The laboratory data, along with the physical condition of the patient, are used by physicians and nurses as the base for their plan of care. Physicians determine doses of medications, frequency and composition of dialysis treatment, and type of diet. If the patient is not taking the medications as prescribed, the amount that is being taken needs to be determined. Any financial stress the patient is having that would prevent purchasing the needed drugs is identified. Referral of the financial problem to the social worker should be done as soon as possible. If the medication is immediately needed for the welfare of the patient, emergency funds might be obtained to purchase them.

Dosages of drugs usually need to be modified. Because patients with CRF are predisposed to a number of other medical problems, they are frequently on multiple medications in addition to the ones used to treat renal-related problems. As a majority of these drugs are excreted, at least in part, by the kidney, the dosage needs to be adjusted. Because of the biochemical and physiologic alterations associated with CRF, the patients often respond to a medication in a different manner than normal individuals. Dialysis may remove substantial amounts of medication. The general classifications of medications that commonly require reduced dosages in patients with CRF include antibacterial agents, analgesics, sedatives, antifungal agents, and cardiac glycosides. Medications that are frequently contraindicated in renal failure include magnesium-containing antacids and laxatives, phosphate-containing enemas, and antibiotics containing potassium.

Nutritional Therapy. The course of CRF may be slowed through intensive nutritional therapy. The main objectives of the therapy are to (1) maintain an optimal nutritional status, (2) prevent protein catabolism, (3) minimize uremic toxicity, (4) stimulate patient well-being, (5) retard progression of renal failure, and (6) postpone initiation of dialysis.[34] To accomplish these goals, the renal failure diet usually includes restriction of protein, fluid, sodium, potassium, and phosphate.

Since CRF patients frequently suffer from anorexia, nausea, vomiting, and diarrhea, consuming adequate nutritional intake is a challenge. Sufficient caloric intake must be provided through carbohydrates and fats (poly- and monounsaturated) to prevent malnutrition (breakdown of body protein) and allow the patient to effectively metabolize the smaller intake of dietary protein.[4] Initially, this may involve the use of total parenteral nutrition (TPN) to furnish essential nutrition.

Protein Restriction. The major breakdown products of both endogenous and exogenous protein (urea, uric acid, sulfate, and organic acids) are nitrogenous and normally excreted by the kidney, but are retained by the patient with renal failure. Prior to dialysis, ideal protein intake should be limited to 0.6 to 0.8 g/kg/day (approximately two to three 2-oz servings of meat). Once dialysis is begun, protein intake may be liberalized to 1 g/kg/day for the patient on hemodialysis and 1.2 to 1.5 g/kg/day for patients undergoing peritoneal dialysis.

In the protein-restricted diet, 65% of the protein intake should be of high biologic value (eggs, meats, and fish) that contains essential amino acids. However, protein from vegetable and dairy sources also contributes to total protein intake.[8] Supplements with essential amino acids are sometimes used to supply all the necessary amino acid building blocks without imposing a burden of nonessential nitrogen-containing compounds when the protein restriction is less than 0.6 g/day.[49] Water-soluble vitamins and folic acid, including oral or IV calcitrol (vitamin D), also are added.

Fluid Restriction. Fluid is usually restricted to an amount equal to the urinary output plus 500 mL to 1 L/day for insensible loss. The amount of insensible loss varies with activity, ambient temperature, and metabolic rate, so the loss must be replaced accordingly. Weight and blood pressure are valuable guides in assisting with regulation of fluid intake. The following foods are also considered to be fluids and therefore must be counted in daily fluid allowances: popsicles, sherbet, syrups or water from canned fruits or vegetables, gelatin (low-quality protein), creamers, pudding, custard, and watermelon.

Sodium and Potassium Restriction. Sodium must be restricted to generally less than 2 to 3 g/day to prevent sodium and water retention. Potassium must be restricted to 2 g or less per day to prevent the development of cardiac arrhythmias and cardiac arrest.[38] It is important to remember that this group of patients cannot use potassium-containing salt substitutes.

Seasonings such as garlic, lemon juice, and vinegar can be used to flavor foods.

Phosphate Restriction. Because the patient with renal failure is unable to excrete normal amounts of phosphate, this substance must be restricted. High levels of phosphate aggravate the hypocalcemia that also develops in renal failure. Foods high in phosphate that should be restricted in renal failure include milk and milk products, meat, fish, poultry, cheese, egg yolks, liver, legumes, whole grain cereals, and nuts.

In addition, patients are generally prescribed aluminum hydroxide antacid preparations that *should be taken at mealtime*. This medication binds with the phosphate in the foods, which is then eliminated through the intestine. Unfortunately, phosphate binders can cause severe constipation, and so stool softeners must frequently be taken. When phosphate levels are normal, calcium carbonate is given at mealtimes to keep the phosphate levels from rising with meals. The aluminum hydroxide is then stopped to prevent aluminum toxicity.

Complications and Prognosis

The incidence of complications from dialysis increases with the age of the patient. These complications are discussed in the section on Dialysis. Patients may also develop problems associated with the uremic syndrome.

Survival is influenced by the age of the patient and medical conditions such as diabetes, arteriosclerotic heart disease, and hypertension. As of 1991, the 1-year survival rate for dialysis patients was 76%.[82]

Nursing Management

The nursing care of a patient with CRF and ESRD is especially complex. Patients not only exhibit the signs and symptoms of the uremic syndrome, but are on complicated medication regimens, must restrict their intake of food and fluid, and must cope with overwhelming psychologic problems related to dialysis and/or transplantation.

The role of nurses in administration of medications and patient education is extremely important. They must be aware of (1) changes in drug therapy that are necessary in renal insufficiency and renal failure, (2) effect of dialysis on drug levels, and (3) common medications that are frequently contraindicated in renal failure. In addition, nurses should be knowledgeable regarding the best circumstances in which to administer medications to facilitate absorption.

The nursing management of the patient with CRF and/or ESRD includes the interventions outlined in Table 47–7 and discussed in this chapter previously. The uremic syndrome predisposes the patients to several serious problems requiring complex nursing management. Care of the patient with the uremic syndrome is discussed in Table 48–11.

Psychologic Stresses. The diagnosis of any life-threatening chronic illness has a profound impact on the patient and

TABLE 48–11

NURSING MANAGEMENT PLAN: THE PATIENT WITH THE UREMIC SYNDROME

Potential Nursing Diagnoses/Collaborative Problems
- *Fluid volume excess related to electrolyte imbalance*
- *Nutrition altered, potential for less than body requirements, related to decreased appetite, retention of toxic metabolites*
- *Impaired gas exchange related to compensatory mechanisms in response to metabolic acidosis or hypoxia*

Goals/Desired Outcomes
- *The patient will remain free of complications. If complications do occur, they will be recognized early and treated promptly.*

Interventions	**Rationale/Significance**
1. Monitor for *fluid imbalances*.	1. Volume overload is a common problem, although volume depletion can also occur.
2. Monitor for *electrolyte* and *acid–base imbalance*. Refer to Table 48–9 related to acute renal failure.	2. Hyperkalemia, hypocalcemia, and hyperphosphatemia are the most common electrolyte abnormalities. Hypermagnesemia can also occur. Metabolic acidosis is present in renal failure.
3. Monitor for *metabolic manifestations*. Instruct the patient in the prescribed diet. Stress the importance of protein intake of high biologic value with dietary parameters. Monitor BUN and creatinine levels, weight and glucose levels, and triglyceride and cholesterol levels.	3. Metabolic abnormalities associated with chronic renal failure include (a) accumulation of end products from protein metabolism, (b) carbohydrate intolerance, and (3) hyperlipidemia.
4. Monitor for the following *neurologic manifestations:* headache, lassitude, changes in mentation, disorientation, and changes in the sleep pattern.	4. The uremic syndrome has several CNS effects.
a. Teach the patient's family about the neurologic effects of the uremic syndrome.	a. The patient's family may become anxious because of neurologic changes.
b. Allow the patient adequate time to think about and respond to discussions.	b. The patient requires more time to process information. The attention span is decreased.
c. Avoid administration of opiates and long-acting barbiturates.	c. Renal excretion or breakdown of medications is decreased.
d. Monitor for the following: numbness and burning in feet, foot drop, tingling of extremities, decreased muscle strength, and change in gait.	d. The uremic syndrome includes several peripheral nervous system effects.
e. Encourage activity.	e. The patient needs to remain as active as possible to maintain strength.
f. Prevent trauma to the legs and feet.	f. The likelihood of trauma is increased because of neurologic deficits.
g. Encourage the patient to change position slowly. Check blood pressure in sitting and standing position (if possible).	g. Autonomic nervous system defects may be present.
5. Monitor for *cardiovascular manifestations* such as hypovolemia and hypertension.	5. Hypervolemia and hypertension are frequent problems for the patient with the uremic syndrome.
a. Assess for symptoms of *pericarditis,* such as tachycardia, ECG changes, a pericardial friction rub (heard best when the patient is sitting up and leaning forward), dyspnea, fever, and chest pain that is relieved by an upright position. Report any symptoms to the physician.	a. The uremic environment inflames the pericardium, so pericarditis is a common complication. A pericardial friction rub is best heard at the left fifth intercostal space during systole.
b. If a pericardiocentesis is needed, assist the physician with the procedure.	
c. If prescribed, administer corticosteroids.	
d. If the patient has been receiving anticoagulants as prescribed, observe closely for signs of pericardial tamponade.	d. Alteration of the pericardial membrane facilitates the collection of fluid in the sac. Bleeding may also occur.
e. Monitor the patient closely for signs of myocardial dysfunction and/or congestive heart failure: dyspnea on exertion, orthopnea, paroxysmal nocturnal dyspnea, chest pain, peripheral edema.	e. Accelerated arteriosclerosis, anemia, and volume overload cause increased workload on the heart.
6. Monitor for *respiratory manifestations*. Monitor the rate, depth, and character of respirations.	6. Tachypnea can occur as a compensatory response to metabolic acidosis or hypoxia.
a. Note the amount and character of sputum.	a. Sputum is thick and tenacious in infection, thin and frothy in pulmonary edema.
b. Monitor for signs and symptoms of pulmonary edema.	b. This condition is discussed in Chap. 21.

Interventions	Rationale/Significance

c. Auscultate the lung fields for the presence of adventitious breath sounds.

d. Instruct the patient to cough and deep breathe.

e. Teach the patient to avoid exposure to persons with colds or influenza.

7. Monitor for *dermatologic manifestations.* Monitor the skin for dryness, signs of scratching, infection, bruising, capillary fragility, poor turgor, and color.

a. Instruct the patient and family in good skin care. Advise to keep nails trimmed, keep skin clean and dry, apply creams or lotions to the skin, and if fluid intake is not restricted, prevent dehydration.

8. Monitor for *GI manifestations.* If present, note the degree of anorexia, nausea, and vomiting.

a. Instruct the patient and family in the prescribed diet.

b. Monitor the serum BUN, potassium, CO_2, and phosphate as indicators of dietary compliance.

c. Inspect the mucous membranes for signs of stomatitis. Encourage the patient to maintain good oral hygiene.

d. Monitor stools and vomitus for gross or occult blood. If they occur, report the findings to the physician.

9. Monitor for *skeletal manifestations.* Monitor serum calcium, phosphate, alkaline phosphatase, and serum parathormone levels.

a. Observe for bone pain, fractures, and muscle weakness.

b. Monitor clinical findings of hypocalcemia: tetany, Chvostek's and Trousseau's signs.

c. Encourage activity and weight bearing, if possible.

d. Teach the patient and family about the effects of hypocalcemia and hyperphosphatemia in CRF.

10. Monitor for *hematologic manifestations.* Observe for the *anemia* of renal failure. Closely monitor the hemoglobin and hematocrit values.

a. Monitor the patient for signs of anemia, such as weakness, dyspnea, tachycardia, palpitations, and pallor.

b. Report initial signs of bleeding to the physician immediately. Monitor the patient for hematemesis, bruises, hemoptysis, and melena.

c. Administer iron, folate, androgen (male hormone) supplements, and erythropoietin as prescribed. Avoid administering iron and phosphate-binding medication at the same time. Administer iron 30 to 60 minutes before meals for best absorption; however, it may also cause stomach irritation.

d. Monitor coagulation studies and platelet counts.

e. Observe the patient for signs and symptoms of infection. A temperature greater than 99°F may be significant.

11. Monitor for *reproductive system* problems. Listen to the patient's concerns. Monitor hormone levels if available. Provide appropriate education.

---

c. Wheezes and crackles indicate pulmonary congestion. A pleural friction rub is associated with uremic pleuritis.

d. Deep breathing aids in expanding alveoli; coughing assists in removing secretions.

e. Uremic patients are more susceptible to respiratory infections than normal.

7. Dry, thin, friable skin develops in patients with uremia. Pruritus is a common problem.

a. Trimmed nails aid in preventing trauma to the skin from scratching. The skin may be dry from decreased oil from sebaceous glands.

8. These are the most common GI symptoms associated with the uremic syndrome.

a. Diet therapy is an important part of therapy.

b. BUN, potassium, and phosphate are increased with dietary indiscretion. Serum CO_2 levels decrease as acidosis increases.

c. The patient is more susceptible to infection.

d. GI bleeding occurs frequently and is related to increased circulating gastrin levels and clotting abnormalities.

9. An increase in alkaline phosphatase occurs in bone destruction.

a. Bone pain and fractures occur in chronic renal failure (CRF). Muscle weakness can occur in CRF.

b. Hypocalcemia is more likely to occur in acute renal failure (ARF). Metabolic acidosis has a protective effect against tetany as it increases the amount of ionized calcium available for muscle use.

c. Weight bearing and exercise may help to prevent bone demineralization.

d. Compliance with the diet and medications can help to prevent renal osteodystrophy.

10. Anemia results from decreased production of erythropoietin. The uremic environment decreases the life span of the RBC.

a. Once the anemia develops, recombinant human erythropoietin may be prescribed to maintain hematocrit around 30%.

b. Bleeding may occur because uremia causes decreased platelet adhesiveness.

c. When iron and phosphate binders are administered together, iron is not absorbed from the GI tract.

d. The patient with uremia usually has a normal platelet count, although it may be slightly reduced in some patients. Coagulation studies should also be normal unless the patient is receiving an anticoagulant.

e. A patient with CRF has a depressed immunologic response to infection.

11. The only successful treatment for these abnormalities is renal transplantation.

family. The development of ESRD in a family member dictates changes in quite literally every facet of life. The manner in which the patient and family adjust to these stresses depends to a great degree on their family system, communication patterns, and preexisting coping patterns. It is helpful to consider the adaptation pattern of the individual patient within the framework described by Reischman and Levy.[63] They described stages through which patients pass as they adjust to dialysis: "honeymoon stage," disenchantment and discouragement, and long-term adaptation.

Patients on dialysis are particularly aware of the possibility of death and physical symptoms just prior to dialysis. Once on dialysis and after they begin feeling better, they may feel particularly happy and hopeful. This *honeymoon stage* may last 6 weeks to 6 months. The *stages of disenchantment and discouragement* that follow may last 3 to 12 months. The patient struggles with the idea of having to depend on treatment for the rest of his or her life and may express feelings of anger, depression, helplessness, or hopelessness. Denial is another common problem associated with this stage. In the final *stage of adaptation,* the patient begins to accept the illness and associated limitations.

Dialysis has impact on both the quantity and the quality of life. Improvements in dialysis and medical management have increased the life expectancy to as much as 20 years or more in some patients. Depending on the patient's

TABLE 48–12

NURSING MANAGEMENT PLAN: ASSISTING THE PATIENT WITH END-STAGE RENAL DISEASE WITH PSYCHOSOCIAL PROBLEMS

Potential Nursing Diagnoses/Collaborative Problems
- Coping, ineffective individual, related to terminal disease
- Grieving, anticipatory, related to nature of terminal disease
- Risk for caregiver role strain related to long-term, ultimately fatal disease

Goals/Desired Outcomes
- The patient will experience minimal psychosocial discomfort.

Interventions	Rationale/Significance
1. Monitor family strengths and weaknesses prior to the onset of the patient's ESRD: family member roles, communication patterns, coping strategies, ways stress is expressed, resources (financial, social, religious). Consult social worker and/or psychologist.	1. The patient is usually a member of a family unit. Responses to discussions will be influenced greatly by preexisting coping strategies and other pertinent patterns associated with family functioning.
2. Encourage open communication between the patient, family, and health care team. • Display a caring attitude. • Use direct eye contact. • Accept feelings of the patient and family. • Encourage family members to openly communicate. • Discuss roles that the patient, family, and health team have in responsibility for management.	2. Frequently, the patient, family, or health care team members may hesitate to express needs, feelings, and reactions. The management of the patient with ESRD necessitates a patient/family/team approach for optimal wellness.
3. Monitor for mood swings, anger, depression, hostility, loss of self-esteem, and denial. • Do not force patient to hear information until he or she is ready to listen. • Acknowledge feelings. • Encourage verbalization. • Spend time with the patient. • Be supportive. • Explore meaning illness has for the patient. Determine how the patient functioned before the illness and how functions will change as a result of the illness.	3. Patient responses vary. Family reaction to patient responses also are variables. It is helpful to determine how the patient perceives the responses of others to himself or herself.
4. Provide patient and family education.	4. This topic is discussed in Table 48–13.
5. Familiarize the patient and family with community resources: social services, National Kidney Foundation, National Association of Patients on Hemodialysis and Transplantation (NAPHT).	5. These patients and their families frequently have multiple needs. The addresses of these organizations are listed in the Patient Education Resources.

age, this information may or may not be consoling. The very nature of the treatment, which includes dialysis, medications, diet, and activity limitations, precipitates stress related to dependency, threat of death, loss of a body function, and frustration related to basic physiologic drives, including hunger, thirst, sleep, and sex.

The patient must constantly change from a "sick role" when dealing with the health care system to a "well role" when dealing with family and society. Roles in the family may need to be changed, causing sexual identity problems. Dependency on a machine may cause body image alterations. Ensuing financial problems may be overwhelming.

Psychosocial Support. Because of the complex treatments prescribed for many patients with renal disorders, psychologic support is needed. Patient and family responses vary dramatically. Nurses must recognize the specific responses of each patient and understand how each patient may adapt to the changes in lifestyle; family and community resources are incorporated to provide additional support for the patient. Table 48–12 contains a plan for the nursing management supporting the psychosocial adjustment of the patient to ESRD.

Patient Teaching. Patient teaching is a critical part of the management of the patient with CRF. Treatment requires a tremendous amount of medical and nursing care and a vast amount of patient and family involvement. Most of the time patients are treated on an outpatient basis so that they are responsible for their own care. A careful teaching plan must be developed to meet each patient's individual needs and to provide information necessary to comply with the requirements of the medical regimen. Patient learning is ongoing and must be evaluated periodically. Table 48–13 contains a teaching plan for these patients.

Patient education is essential *before* a patient begins dialysis. Certain points need to be considered:

- If the patient is uremic and will eventually begin dialysis, enlist the help of the dialysis team in providing information about this treatment at the appropriate time. The procedure should be briefly explained, including the venipuncture attachment to the artificial kidney and how the blood is returned to the patient.
- If there is a chapter of the National Association of Patients on Hemodialysis and Transplantation (NAPHT) in or near your community and it seems the patient would benefit from a visit with another patient on dialysis, arrange the visit while the patient is still in the hospital.
- As it is of utmost importance to maintain autonomy at the onset of the demanding regimen of dialysis, the patient must be taught that one can still function well with this chronic illness and not be an invalid. Of course, health care professionals provide care when the patient is acutely ill.

TABLE 48–13

TEACHING PLAN: THE PATIENT WITH END-STAGE RENAL DISEASE AND THE PATIENT'S FAMILY

Teaching Principles	Rationale/Significance
1. Explain normal kidney function, including anatomy; urine formation and fluid, electrolyte, acid–base balance; and production of renin; erythropoietin, and the active form of vitamin D.	1. The patient and family will achieve a better understanding of the disease process if they are familiar with normal kidney function.
2. Give cause of kidney failure and potential problems associated with the uremic syndrome.	2. The patient and family should be very familiar with the signs and symptoms to report (listed in Table 48–11).
3. Describe fluid retention in renal failure: weight gain, edema, shortness of breath, hypertension (instruct patient how to check blood pressure).	3. This is discussed in the section on hypervolemia in Table 47–7.
4. Explain significance of laboratory tests, including normal values and dialysis normals: BUN and its relationship to protein intake; creatinine; sodium, potassium, phosphate, and calcium; hematocrit.	4. The patient and family should be able to follow and understand progress and/or changes reflected in laboratory tests.
5. Give dietary restrictions: protein, potassium, sodium, phosphate.	5. Compliance with the diet helps the patient to feel as well as possible and avoid complications.
6. Describe medications: name, dose, frequency, and side effects. The patient should carry a list of all medications in wallet in the event of an emergency and also wear a Medic-Alert bracelet or necklace.	6. Compliance with medications will usually enhance the patient's physical status.
7. Explain dialysis; definition, types, advantages of each type, vascular access.	7. The patient and family should have input into the type of dialysis selected (discussed in section on Dialysis). Information should be provided before dialysis is initiated, if possible.
8. Discuss transplantation.	8. This topic is discussed in the section on Transplantation.

• Remember that when treatment is initiated during convalescence, the patient will usually provide clues indicating readiness for more independence.

Community Care

The community care of a patient with CRF is particularly challenging. The patient and family need continued psychologic support and educational reinforcement of information related to diet, medications, and dialysis (if required). The activities of various social agencies need to be coordinated to adequately address financial, transportation, and other types of problems frequently encountered. In addition, the nurse must constantly assess the patient thoroughly for the multiple physical complications associated with CRF.

Evaluation/Desired Outcomes: Chronic Renal Failure. The patient (or with the family's assistance) will:

1. Verbalize information related to dietary restrictions and demonstrate dietary compliance
2. Verbalize the name, dose, action, frequency, and side effects of all medications and demonstrate medication compliance
3. Comply with dialysis regimen, if indicated
4. Keep scheduled appointments for follow-up
5. Achieve a lifestyle compatible with the physical condition and incorporate those changes necessary for health and well-being

■ DIALYSIS

Dialysis refers to the diffusion of solutes through a semipermeable membrane that separates two solutions. Hemodialysis and peritoneal dialysis are two forms used clinically to correct many of the abnormalities of blood composition that result from acute or chronic renal failure.

• *Hemodialysis* refers to the flow of a patient's blood from a vascular access through a catheter and tubing to an "artificial kidney." Metabolic waste products plus excessive electrolytes and fluid are removed from the blood as they diffuse into a special fluid called a dialysate (discussed later) in the artificial kidney. The cleansed blood is then returned through tubing and a catheter to a patient's vein.
• *Peritoneal dialysis* refers to the instillation of dialysate into a patient's peritoneal cavity. Through the process of dialysis, the excessive metabolic waste products plus excessive electrolytes and fluid move from the capillaries in the peritoneal membrane into the dialysate; then the dialysate is drained from the peritoneal cavity.

Both forms of treatment may be used either temporarily until the patient regains kidney function or chronically to sustain life in the person with ESRD.

Goals

The four basic goals of dialysis therapy when the patient has renal failure are to:

• Remove excess end products of protein metabolism, such as urea and creatinine, from the blood
• Maintain safe concentrations of serum electrolytes, such as potassium
• Remove excess fluid from the body
• Correct acidosis and aid in replacement of the blood's bicarbonate buffer system

Dialysis can also be used to remove some excessive drugs, which may be taken accidentally or in a suicide attempt.

Principles of Dialysis

The key concepts related to dialysis include the physical principles of diffusion, filtration, and osmosis. These forces move solutes and water across a semipermeable membrane between two solutions. In dialysis, the semipermeable membrane is either an artificial membrane (for hemodialysis) or the patient's own peritoneal membrane (for peritoneal dialysis).

Dialysate. The solution used on the opposite side of the membrane to the blood is a specially prepared electrolyte solution called the *dialysate* or *bath*. Dialysate contains important electrolytes in varying concentrations, which prevents their excessive removal. It also contains acid buffers, which are absorbed into the bloodstream. These substances assist in correcting the metabolic acidosis present in renal failure. The difference in concentration of substances in the dialysate and the patient's blood controls the amount and direction of movement across the semipermeable membrane of wastes and other substances. The components of dialysate for hemodialysis and peritoneal dialysis are listed in Table 48–14.

Factors Affecting Movement of Solutes and Water. *Diffusion* refers to the movement of a solute from an area of higher concentration to an area of lower concentration across a semipermeable membrane. The ions normally present in the blood and in the dialysate diffuse in both directions and reach an equilibrium. Factors affecting diffusion of particles include the molecular size of the particles, the pore size of the membrane, and the concentration of the solute on the two sides of the membrane. The large size of the red blood cells and white blood cells (and proteins in hemodialysis) prevents them from passing through the small pores in the semipermeable membrane. Urea, creatinine, and other substances are small enough to diffuse from the blood into the dialysate. If the blood is deficient in a substance, such as bicarbonate, a higher concentration of this substance in the dialysate will cause it to move into the blood, raising the blood level.

Osmosis refers to movement of water molecules to equalize their concentration on the two sides of a semipermeable membrane. The *osmotic gradient* causes water mol-

TABLE 48-14

COMPONENTS OF DIALYSATE

	Hemodialysate	Peritoneal Dialysate
Sodium	130 to 135	140 to 141
Calcium	2.5 to 3.5	3.5
Magnesium	0.5 to 1.0	0.5 to 1.5
Potassium	0 to 2.0	0 to 4
Chloride	100 to 119	96 to 102
Acetate	32 to 38	
Lactate		35 to 40
Bicarbonate	30 to 38	
Glucose	1 to 200 mg/dL	
Dextrose		
1.5%		15 g/L
4.25%		42.5 g/L

Note: All substances are in mEq/L unless stated otherwise.
(Source: *Daugiradis and Ing.*[20])

ecules to move to the side with the higher concentration of solutes. In peritoneal dialysis, dextrose in the dialysate creates an osmotic gradient that causes water molecules to move from the vessels into the peritoneal cavity.

Filtration is the movement of solutes and water through a semipermeable membrane by hydrostatic pressure. *Hydrostatic pressure* refers to the pressure within a closed system, such as that exerted against the wall of a vessel by the fluid within the vessel. Hydrostatic pressure results from pressure gradients. Filtration represents a minor mechanism for solute removal in both hemodialysis and peritoneal dialysis.

Three additional factors affect the movement of solutes and water. The *temperature of the solution* modifies the rate of diffusion and osmosis. As the temperature increases, the rate of diffusion and osmosis increases. The *rate of blood flow* influences the rate of exchange on one side of the membrane. The *time of contact* of the two solutions through a semipermeable membrane affects the concentration: the longer the contact, the more the solutions will become alike in their concentrations of the substances that move through the pores; the shorter the contact time, the less the solutions become alike.

HEMODIALYSIS

Hemodialysis, treatment with an *artificial kidney,* is a process that cleanses the blood of accumulated waste products when the normal functioning of the kidney stops during acute or chronic failure. Artificial kidneys operate outside the patient's body and, thus, heparinization is required.

As the patient's blood passes through the artificial kidney, waste products, excessive electrolytes, and water are removed. A tolerable chemical equilibrium can be maintained for several days between treatments. The hemodialysis system is represented in Fig. 48–3.

Access

A reliable access to the circulation is essential to perform hemodialysis, because blood must be removed through an artery and returned through a vein to the patient at a rapid rate (approximately 250 to 500 mL/min). Arteries could provide adequate blood flow, but they are deep vessels and difficult to enter by puncture. Peripheral veins are close to the skin surface and are easy to enter by puncture, but they do not have the pressure that would supply the rapid blood flow needed. Therefore, surgical modifications are frequently made to increase the flow needed.

Vascular Accesses. Vascular accesses provide a passageway to the blood supply in amounts necessary for effective hemodialysis. They can be divided into external and internal types. Figure 48–4 illustrates the various types.

External Vascular Accesses. External vascular accesses include arteriovenous (AV) shunts and catheters. To create an AV shunt, cannulas are placed in an artery and adjacent vein and then they are joined externally (Fig. 48–4A). During hemodialysis, blood flows from the artery to the dialyzer, then to the vein. The shunt can be used immediately after insertion. This type of access may be used for performing slow, continuous therapies such as continuous arteriovenous hemofiltration (CAV-H).[20]

A *subclavian* or *internal jugular venous double-lumen catheter* may be used immediately and can be left in place several weeks.[20] The catheter is often placed at the same time as an AV fistula or graft is performed, and the catheter

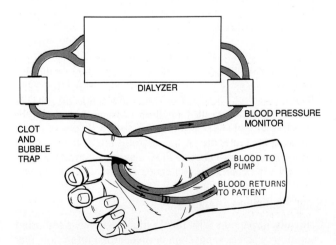

Figure 48–3. Hemodialysis system. Access to the circulation is illustrated as blood flowing from an artery to the dialyzer and returning to the body through a vein. (*Adapted from Ahrens.*[2])

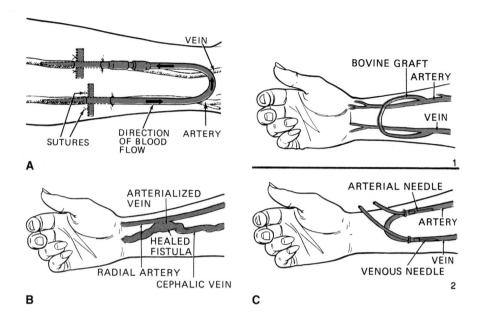

Figure 48–4. Vascular accesses. **A.** External arteriovenous shunt with a silicone cannula. **B.** Anastomosis to form arteriovenous fistula. **C.** (**1**) Bovine graft in place and (**2**) placement of needles in graft for hemodialysis. (*From Ahrens.*[2])

is used until the fistula or graft heals. Complications of placement include puncture of the lungs and puncture of surrounding arteries and veins. After removal, stenosis of the subclavian vein at the site of insertion can cause venous obstruction and severe edema of the arm. A femoral catheter may be used for acute care.

Internal Vascular Accesses. Internal angioaccesses include an AV fistula and an AV graft (Fig. 48–4B and C).

An *AV fistula* is created by the surgical anastomosis of an artery and a vein so that a large amount of blood from the artery flows directly into the vein through the fistula and enlarges the vein. Needles can then be placed in the area for access to both an artery and a vein. The fistula should mature in 4 to 6 weeks to permit healing and the development of adequate blood flow. The large blood volume usually causes the elastic vein and its branches to dilate. The turbulent blood flow produces a palpable vibration known as a *thrill;* it is called a *bruit* when audible with a stethoscope.

An *AV graft* is an artificial vessel surgically implanted subcutaneously into an arm or a leg. One end is anastomosed to a large artery and the other end to a large vein. The arterial blood is shunted through the graft and into the vein. An AV graft is used in those patients whose peripheral veins are not suitable for an AV fistula. Types of materials used for grafts are bovine (carotid artery from a cow) or polytetrafluoroethylene (PTFE, a synthetic graft). A portion of the patient's own saphenous vein may also be used.

Slow, Continuous Therapies

Critically ill patients with renal failure may have comorbid conditions, such as septicemia or myocardial infarction, that cause them to be hemodynamically unstable. The susceptibility to hypotension often makes treatment with intermittent hemodialysis difficult. Therefore, a slow, continuous

therapy such as *continuous arteriovenous hemofiltration* (CAV-H) or *continuous arteriovenous hemodialysis* (CAV-HD) are prescribed. In these procedures, a shunt may provide blood access but other types of catheters are more frequently used. Arterial blood flows through a catheter to a small blood filter and then back to the patient's vein through another catheter. The patient's own blood pressure propels the blood through this circuit. During these procedures, varying amounts of fluid and waste products are slowly and continuously removed. The processes may be used for prolonged periods of time (several days).[60,72,75]

Care of the Patient Undergoing Hemodialysis

Hemodialysis is a technical procedure that requires excellent aseptic technique and a basic understanding of electrical and mechanical dynamics. It also requires keen skills of observation, assessment, and problem solving and a thorough understanding of the entire treatment regimen for each patient, including laboratory data, medications, diet, and prescribed dialysis therapy.

The nurses' roles in the dialysis setting are multifaceted. Dialysis nurses must have a thorough understanding of the technical aspects of treatment to effectively supervise the care given by other dialysis personnel. They must have a thorough understanding of the following procedures: preparing the dialyzer for the patient, predialysis physical assessment, venipuncture, initiation of dialysis, monitoring during dialysis, terminating dialysis, and postdialysis physical assessment. They must also be able to look beyond the routine work related to dialysis to see each patient as an individual with special needs.

During *predialysis nursing management,* the patient is advised about adjustment of medications. Blood pressure medications are frequently withheld for 6 to 12 hours prior to hemodialysis to facilitate the patient's hemodynamic tolerances of fluid removal. Water-soluble vitamins are preferably given after dialysis treatments. Patients are usually more comfortable and tolerate dialysis better if they eat before the treatment. Dialysis takes 2 to 5 hours and patients are usually not permitted to eat while being dialyzed, and so they can become extremely hungry.

Immediately prior to hemodialysis, the nurse performs the following assessments: (1) vital signs; (2) weight and its comparison with the postdialysis weight from the last treatment to identify net fluid gain or loss; (3) fluid assessment (weight, blood pressure, examination of neck veins for engorgement, and checking for edema); (4) chest assessment; (5) vascular access (described above); (6) findings indicating electrolyte imbalance; (7) assistance in determining anticoagulation needs; (8) neurologic and psychologic assessment; and (10) educational needs.

The responsibilities for *nursing management during dialysis* are performed by trained dialysis staff. The nurse performs the following: (1) collects all required blood samples at the time of hookup but before dialysis has started (the dialysis procedure alters serum electrolytes quickly so that blood samples taken during dialysis do not reflect accurate levels of many substances); (2) monitors all equipment; (3) continually monitors the patient for possible complications (excessive fluid removal, electrolyte changes, pyrogenic reactions, and bleeding); and (4) observes for signs of emotional distress.

The following are included in *postdialysis nursing management:* (1) assists the patient into a restful position; (2) observes the vascular access for hematoma formation, obvious bleeding (if present, applies firm pressure), and patency by presence of thrill and bruit; (3) observes for other sources of bleeding, such as epistaxis or from the GI or urinary tracts; (4) monitors the blood pressure; (5) reports unusually low or high readings for the individual patient and administers prescribed medications; (6) monitors the temperature; (7) offers the patient food allowed on his or her dietary prescription; and (8) reviews the patient's dialysis record.

In patients with a *femoral, internal jugular,* or *subclavian catheter,* the nurse should:

1. Observe the site every shift to note signs of infection or bleeding

2. Perform site care, usually done at the time of dialysis, using aseptic technique

3. Monitor the pulse, capillary filling, and presence or absence of edema in the distal extremity

4. If bleeding occurs or the catheter becomes dislodged, apply pressure and notify the physician immediately

Patient Education

It is important to teach the patients how the vascular access was surgically created so that they have a more thorough understanding of the self-care necessary to maintain it. The following information needs to be included for *internal* vascular accesses:

1. Avoid tight clothing around the access that may decrease the blood flow and cause clotting.

2. Check the access routinely (at least two times daily) for the "buzz" that indicates adequate blood flow. If it becomes difficult to palpate or does not "buzz," notify the physician immediately, as the access may be clotted. In addition, notify the physician if there is anything unusual about the access, such as redness, swelling, drainage, and pain.

3. Watch the vascular access frequently after treatment, noting any signs of swelling, infection, or obvious bleeding. Should the puncture sites start bleeding again, apply firm pressure to them, and call for help immediately because a great deal of blood may be lost in a short period.

4. Do not allow anyone to take blood pressures or withdraw blood from an extremity with an access.

5. Do not sleep with pressure on the extremity with the access.

6. Avoid the use of creams or lotions over the access site.

Patients with *external* vascular access (shunt or subclavian or jugular catheter) should also do the following.

1. For a shunt, always keep a pair of bulldog clamps (small, strong clamps) attached to the dressing. Practice using the clamps. Should the tubing become disconnected, use the bulldog clamps immediately and clamp both the arterial and venous cannulas. Call the physician immediately.

2. Periodically watch the color of the blood in the shunt tubing. If the blood turns dark, call the physician because it may be clotted.

3. Do not do any physical activity that might dislodge the access accidentally.

4. Call the physician if a fever or other signs of infection develop.

5. Protect the access while bathing by preventing it from becoming wet in the water. It can be wrapped in plastic wrap for protection.

PERITONEAL DIALYSIS

In peritoneal dialysis, the semipermeable membrane used is the patient's capillaries in the peritoneal membrane of the abdominal cavity. The procedure involves the instillation of dialysate into the peritoneal cavity, allowing time for substance exchange, and then removal of the dialysate. This simple procedure is used in ARF, CRF, poisoning, and edematous and acidotic states.

Peritoneal dialysis is frequently used to sustain life in the patient with CRF who is being evaluated for chronic hemodialysis or transplantation or waiting for the vascular access to mature to begin hemodialysis. It is a safe method of treatment for patients with (1) bleeding problems who cannot receive the heparin required during hemodialysis, (2) severe cardiovascular disease who cannot tolerate rapid fluid removal, (3) severe vascular access problems, and (4) diabetics who cannot tolerate hemodialysis.

Relative *contraindications* to peritoneal dialysis include recent abdominal surgery, paralytic ileus, bowel distention, diffuse intra-abdominal adhesions, an open drain-ing wound (because of the possibility of contamination from the wound), or a severe malnourished hypoproteine-mic state. It may be used in several of these situations if hemodialysis is *absolutely* contraindicated. It is *not* the treatment of choice when rapid correction of imbalances is indicated because the clearance of certain toxins is much slower than with hemodialysis.

Advantages of this technique are the relative ease; it can be used in hospitals without the sophisticated equipment needed for hemodialysis and it can also be used in the home. A disadvantage is that it is very time consuming. A higher-protein diet must be consumed because, unlike with hemodialysis, significant amounts of protein are lost in the dialysate.

Procedure for Peritoneal Dialysis for an Acute Condition

1. Percutaneous placement of a catheter into the peritoneal cavity (Fig. 48–5). A temporary catheter may be placed by puncture of the abdominal wall. Complications include puncture of the intestines or bladder or one of several major arteries and veins. A permanent type of peritoneal catheter may be used for acute or chronic dialysis.

2. Instillation of dialysate (usually 2 L) into the cavity (*in-flow*).

3. Movement of metabolic wastes, electrolytes, and water by diffusion, filtration, and osmosis (*dwell time*).

4. Drainage of the altered dialysate from the peritoneal cavity (*outflow*).

Figure 48–5 diagrams peritoneal dialysis, showing placement of the catheter as it is attached to inflow and outflow lines. Table 48–15 describes the nursing management for an acutely ill patient needing peritoneal dialysis.

Home Peritoneal Dialysis. Home peritoneal dialysis is a simple technique to teach and learn. The three types do not require a partner or a vascular access, both of which are needed with home hemodialysis.

In daily *continuous cyclic peritoneal dialysis* (CCPD), an automated peritoneal dialysis machine allows the patient to sleep during dialysis while it delivers sterile dialysate, allowing variable periods for inflow time, dwell time, and outflow time. Volume and temperature parameters are monitored, and alarms are activated when limits are violated. Fluid may also be left in the abdominal cavity during the day and drained at night.

Continuous ambulatory peritoneal dialysis (CAPD) usually involves three to four exchanges of 2 L each in 24 hours and dwell times of 4 to 10 hours. A dialysate bag is connected to a permanent peritoneal catheter at all times. The patient attaches a full bag, controls the inflow and dwell times, and then lowers the bag to collect the outflow. The procedure is then repeated. CAPD avoids machinery, is a relatively simple technique, permits a more normal food and fluid intake, and provides more opportunity for the patient to return to normal activities. The patient's personal

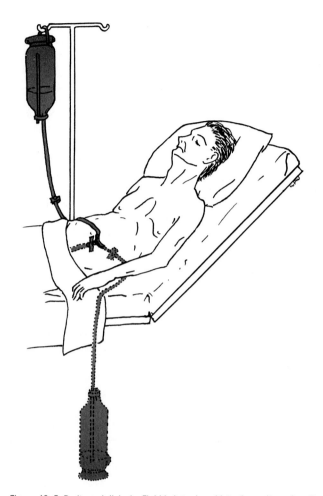

Figure 48–5. Peritoneal dialysis. Fluid is introduced into the peritoneal cavity through tubing and a catheter, time is allowed for substance exchange, then the fluid drains when the bottle is lowered (or there may be a separate drainage system).

hygiene and home environment must be clean to prevent peritonitis. The continuous presence of the catheter in the abdomen may be distressful to some patients.

With the commonly used *chronic intermittent peritoneal dialysis* (CIPD), dialysis may be done three to five times a week for 10 to 12 hours. The total weekly dialysis time varies from 30 to 60 hours according to the patient's condition. A stable, supportive home environment is important.

Evaluation/Desired Outcomes: Hemodialysis or Peritoneal Dialysis. The patient will:

1. Achieve satisfactory fluid, electrolyte, and acid–base balance

2. Experience no or minimal complications or side effects of the dialysis procedure

3. (Along with the family) understand the disease, the treatment, and other pertinent information related to maintaining health and safety

TABLE 48-15

NURSING MANAGEMENT PLAN: AN ACUTELY ILL PATIENT NEEDING PERITONEAL DIALYSIS

Potential Nursing Diagnoses/Collaborative Problems
- *Infection, risk for, related to invasive procedure and immunosuppression*
- *Altered nutrition, potential for more than body requirements related to false assurance of the effects of the dialysis*
- *Knowledge deficit related to implementing procedure, diet modifications, complications of therapy*

Goals/Desired Outcomes
- *The patient will have waste products of protein metabolism, excessive electrolytes, excessive nonvolatile acids, and/or toxic drugs adequately removed from the blood and will experience no complications.*

Interventions	Rationale/Significance
1. Weigh the patient and check the vital signs.	1. Baseline data are needed.
2. To assist with *introduction of the peritoneal catheter* (which is done at the bedside): a. Instruct the patient to empty the bladder. b. Shave and cleanse the area from the umbilicus to the symphysis pubis for the insertion of the trocar about 1 to 2 in. below the umbilicus.	2. a. If distended, the bladder may be perforated by the trocar. b. After the skin is anesthetized, a small incision is made into the skin by the physician. A trocar (a sharply pointed instrument contained in a metal cannula) is inserted into the peritoneal cavity. The trocar is then removed, leaving in place the cannula through which the catheter is advanced in the cavity; then the cannula is removed. If a permanent catheter is placed, a small surgical procedure is required.
c. After the catheter is sutured in place, assist with connecting the catheter to the dialysis inflow and outflow tubings. *Using strict aseptic technique,* attach the bottles of previously warmed dialysate to the catheter.	c. Aseptic technique is used to prevent peritonitis. The solution is warmed to prevent the patient from becoming chilled and to speed the exchange.
3. For the *inflow* (about 5 to 10 minutes), clamp the outflow tubing and unclamp the inflow tubing. Allow the fluid to flow in slowly. Assess the patient for abdominal discomfort.	3. Two liters of solution are generally used for each cycle in an adult. The fluid flows in by gravity. Antibiotics, insulin, or heparin may be added to the dialysate. Xylocaine can be added to decrease pain associated with the inflow.
4. During the *dwell time* (15 to 45 minutes), clamp the inflow tubing as soon as the fluid bottle is empty.	4. The rate of solute exchange is affected by the concentration gradient, surface area of the peritoneum, temperature of the solution, and duration of dwell time.
5. During the *outflow time* (20 to 30 minutes), unclamp the outflow tubing while maintaining closure of the inflow clamp. Collect the drained dialysis fluid in a container beside the bedside and carefully measure it. If there is a problem with drainage, assist the patient to turn, change positions, and gently massage his or her abdomen.	5. The dialysate should be clear and pale yellow, although it may be bloody initially.
6. Repeat steps 3 through 5 for the number of exchanges prescribed by the physician.	6. Each outflow should be about 100 to 200 mL more than inflow except for the first cycle (which may be more) and possibly the last cycle (which may be less).
7. Monitor the patient's temperature, pulse, respiration, and blood pressure throughout the procedure. Monitor the patient's weight once or twice daily. Observe for muscle cramps, which can occur with rapid fluid removal.	7. A spiking temperature and increased pulse and respiration may indicate peritonitis, which is a potential complication of peritoneal dialysis. As fluid is removed, the BP will decrease. If fluid is retained, overload may occur.
8. Monitor the patient for complications: a. *Peritonitis* causes abdominal pain, cloudy fluid, fever, nausea, and vomiting. Send a sample of outflow fluid for culture and cell count. b. *Pain* can be caused by peritonitis. If caused by sensitivity to the peritoneal dialysate on inflow, decrease the rate of inflow. If the patient experiences *shoulder pain,* explain that this is caused by the diaphragm being irritated; elevate the head of the bed.	8. a. Peritonitis is a common complication, especially when a temporary catheter is used. It is removed as soon as the dialysis has been completed. b. See item 8a. The shoulder pain, which is caused by diaphragmatic irritation, is called *Kehr's sign.*

(Continued)

TABLE 48–15   (*Continued*)

NURSING MANAGEMENT PLAN: AN ACUTELY ILL PATIENT NEEDING PERITONEAL DIALYSIS

Interventions	Rationale/Significance
c. *Shortness of breath* may be improved by elevating the head of the bed. Encourage the patient to cough and deep breathe.	c. Shortness of breath is caused by elevation of the diaphragm. The patient is at risk for pneumonia and atelectasis secondary to decreased lung expansion.
d. *Bleeding* at the abdominal site or intra-abdominally. Monitor the hematocrit closely.	d. Some bleeding usually occurs related to placement of the catheter, but this should progressively clear.
e. Watery *diarrhea* or sudden increase in "urine output."	e. These may indicate bowel or bladder puncture.
f. *Infection* at the site, producing redness, bleeding, drainage, and swelling of the site or catheter tunnel. Keep the site dry. Use aseptic techniques for dressing changes.	f. Infections at the site occur more commonly if there is leakage of fluid from the peritoneal cavity.
g. Hyperglycemia.	g. Diabetics may become hyperglycemic from the dextrose in the dialysate. Insulin can be added to the dialysate.
9. Carefully record the amounts of inflow and outflow, as well as other forms of intake and output (usually a special dialysis record is available). Contact the physician if the outflow is greater than 500 mL (or the mL stated by the physician) in excess of the amount instilled.	9. The physician may change the inflow or dwell time. To prevent hypovolemia in some patients who are not edematous (such as those requiring dialysis because of a drug overdose), some physicians prescribe that the outflow tubing be clamped when a certain amount of dialysate has drained.
10. Contact the physician if the patient is retaining the peritoneal dialysate.	10. The physician is usually contacted if the patient has retained more than 250 mL, because glucose absorption may become a problem.

■ RENAL TRANSPLANTATION

The first successful human kidney transplant was performed in Boston in 1954;[10] the donor and recipient were identical twins. Since that time kidney transplantation has become a commonly accepted form of treatment for patients with ESRD.

Criteria for Kidney Transplantation

Patients with ESRD and their families should understand the options available: hemodialysis, peritoneal dialysis, renal transplantation, or death without treatment. The risks, benefits, and complications of each treatment should be discussed. The sooner this information is presented, the more time the patient will have to consider each modality with the type of accompanying lifestyle changes. The final choice should be made by the patient, who must understand that there are no guarantees with the transplant procedure and also the possible adverse side effects from drugs used after transplantation. It may be difficult for the patient to accept this uncertainty in his or her life.

Not every patient is a suitable transplant candidate. The patient's age, psychologic status, and general health need to be evaluated. One of the most important criteria is a fully informed and motivated patient who wishes to try transplantation.

The decision to seriously consider a patient for transplantation may be influenced by the primary disease process. Diabetes mellitus, systemic lupus erythematosus, and localized or systemic infections are examples of disease

processes that require further evaluation, although increasing numbers of diabetics are receiving transplants. The patient must be currently free of any type of malignancy, which gives the patient with a history of treated cancer a chance to be a candidate.

Immunology

A complex problem is caused by the unanswered questions concerning the immune system, because a person is receiving foreign antigens when a kidney is received. The body recognizes these antigens as different from its own and activates its immune system. Lymphocytes and antibodies are produced that can destroy the foreign antigen—the kidney—resulting in rejection.

Genetic information is inherited from each parent (haplotype). The total genetic information is the *phenotype*. The concept of inheritance of genes is shown here with four antigens.

MOTHER						FATHER
*0			CHILDREN			#%
	*#	*%	0#	0%	*#	
	A	B	C	D	E	
Identical match:		Exactly the same antigens inherited				(Siblings A and E)
One haplotype match:		Half the same antigens inherited				(Siblings A and B, A and C, B and D, B and E, C and D, C and E)
Mismatch:		Totally dissimilar antigens inherited				(Siblings A and D)

Histocompatibility Testing. Histocompatibility testing measures the degree of antigenic compatibility between the donor and recipient. Selection of the most histocompatible donor is done to avoid rejection. Important antigens to assess are located on the surfaces of white blood cells and nucleated cells of most body tissues. All these tests can be done on peripheral blood samples. Following are the standard tests that are used.[34]

- *ABO.* To identify a person's blood type (A, B, AB, or O). The Rh factor is not important unless the recipient will be receiving blood transfusions from the donor. Compatibility between the ABO blood groups of the donor and recipient is an absolute requirement for transplantation.
- *Human leukocyte antigen (HLA) typing.* To identify known human leukocyte antigens of both the donor and the recipient.
- *White cell cross-match test for preformed antibodies.* To determine whether the recipient has formed antibodies to the donor tissue antigens. If the test is positive, the transplant procedure cannot be performed because the organ would be rejected quickly. Patients on maintenance hemodialysis are exposed to various forms of antigenic stimulation that may occur during blood transfusions or certain viral or bacterial infections. These patients develop antibodies to the lymphocytes of a certain portion of the general population.
- *Mixed lymphocyte culture.* To demonstrate the responsiveness of the recipient to the donor cells. Lymphocytes from the donor and recipient are maintained in tissue culture medium for 5 days. A high level of responsiveness has been demonstrated to correlate with poor graft survival. This culture is done with living related donors.

Potential Donors

The two main types of kidney donors are living related and cadaver. Federal reimbursement pays the medical expenses associated with organ donation of kidneys as a part of Medicare.

Living Related Donors. The category of eligible donors includes members of the immediate family (blood related); occasionally non–blood related donors are used. There are several advantages to receiving a living related kidney as opposed to a cadaveric kidney: (1) more time is available for histocompatibility testing; (2) organs tend to be similar to the patient's tissues and generally survive for a longer period; (3) less immunosuppressive medication may be needed because of the similarity in tissues; (4) fewer complications may develop; and (5) surgery can be planned more conveniently.

Asking a family member to donate an organ can be a difficult task for the patient. Some patients will not ask even though they have a close family relationship. Prior negative family experiences, such as sibling rivalry, may prevent the patient from asking for a kidney.

All potential donors must understand that there is a surgical risk (even though very small) associated with the donation procedure and that there is no guarantee that the transplant will be successful. It is important that the motivation of the donor be sincerely altruistic and that there are no known attempts at coercion.[58]

If family members voice their willingness to be considered as donors, extensive preliminary testing and evaluation are scheduled to identify potential donors. Different blood types alone may eliminate willing potential donors. A complete physical examination including blood, urine, chest x-ray, ECG, and renal studies is performed on a potential donor. If all potential donors are eliminated during the workup, the patient needs to decide if he or she wants to be placed on the waiting list to receive a cadaveric organ.

Cadaver Donors. Healthy individuals who suffer a fatal accident or a rapidly progressive terminal illness are the major sources of cadaver kidneys. Cadaver kidneys are usually taken from subjects who die from irreversible brain damage; normally both kidneys are removed. Organs obtained from a cadaveric donor can be kept viable for up to 48 hours by use of the hypothermic perfusion machine.[58] During this time the United Network of Organ Sharing (UNOS) quickly identifies the best matched recipient through computerized histocompatibility information, and preoperative preparation is done while the kidney is being transported to the appropriate location.

Preoperative Preparation

Preoperative preparation of a patient receiving a transplant from a living related donor is extensive. The physician discusses the following with the patient and family at least 1 month prior to surgery: surgical procedure, medications and their side effects, possible complications, meaning of rejection, expected outcome of surgery, and expected length of hospitalization. A detailed physical examination and laboratory and radiographic studies are performed on the recipient. The most common cause of recipient morbidity and mortality after transplantation is sepsis. Something as seemingly minor as tooth decay can cause trouble.[34]

The potential recipient will be dialyzed within 24 hours of surgery. The patient must understand that postoperative dialysis is common and should be expected. The donor's operation is more extensive than the recipient's and the donor may experience more pain postoperatively than the recipient because of the retroperitoneal location of the kidney.

Surgery

The donor kidney is placed in the lower quadrant of the abdomen outside the peritoneal cavity (Fig. 48–6). The renal artery and renal vein are anastomosed to the corresponding iliac vessels and the donor ureter is tunneled into the bladder. The peritoneal cavity is not entered, leaving the kidney fairly close to the surface.

Complications. After surgery, the recipient needs to be observed for complications. These include rejection (discussed next), infection, and renal failure. Complications of

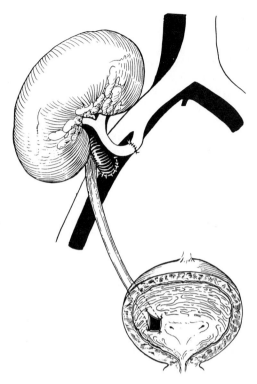

Figure 48–6. Renal transplantation (anastomoses to internal iliac artery, iliac vein, and bladder). (*From Tanagho and McAninch.[79]*)

retroperitoneal bleeding, arterial stenosis, and urine leakage into the pelvic cavity require surgical repair.

Rejection. Rejection is the major complication. The normal fate of renal transplantation from one individual to another (with the exception of identical twins) is inevitable rejection; it may occur immediately after surgery or develop over a period of years. Rejection is an immunologic attack against the foreign donor organ in an attempt to get rid of it. The reaction is stimulated by foreign histocompatibility antigens. Three major types of rejection are hyperacute, acute, and chronic.

Hyperacute rejection (1) is irreversible, (2) occurs minutes to 48 hours posttransplantation, (3) is a humoral immune response, (4) results in graft destruction, (5) does not respond to treatment, and (6) necessitates removal of the transplanted kidney.

Acute rejection, a cellular immune response, is common and usually develops within the first weeks to a year of transplantation. *Clinical findings* include fever, hypertension, weight gain, lethargy, elevated WBCs, graft tenderness and swelling, significant reduction in urine volume, and increased serum creatinine levels. Early diagnosis of rejection is essential. *Treatment* with prompt administration of immunosuppressive agents, radiation therapy, or both may reverse declining renal function and prevent irreversible damage.[18,34]

Chronic rejection is believed to be both a cellular and a humoral immune response. It is a slow process that ultimately results in destruction of the transplanted kidney. Because of its insidious nature, clinical findings may be absent, but deterioration of renal function will be noted in blood and urine analyses. No treatment for this type of rejection is available. Transplants that undergo chronic rejection may be left in place.

Immunosuppressive medications used in the clinical management of the patient include prednisone, cyclophosphamide (Cytoxan), cyclosporine (Sandimmune), and azathioprine (Imuran). Antilymphocyte globulin and antithymocyte globulin may also be administered.

Long-term Complications. The multiple complications that may develop include (1) rejection, (2) infection, (3) renal failure, (4) recurrence of the original kidney disease, (5) complications as a result of drug therapy, (6) GI ulcers and bleeding, (7) increased risk of cancer of the skin, cervix, and lymphoid tissue, (8) osteoporosis, (9) hypertension, and (10) steroid-induced diabetes mellitus. The changes in physical appearance (obesity, cushingoid appearance, and acne) are particularly difficult for young adults.

Prognosis. The prognosis depends on the reason for the transplant, other disorders, and the complications listed above. The expected national success rate for a living related transplant after 1 year is 90 to 95%. The cadaveric kidney transplant success rate at 1 year is 75 to 85%.[19] Although 1- and 2-year graft survival rates have improved over the past decade, the patient usually faces declining graft functions at about 5 years.[10] However, in a follow-up *research study* of 14 patients with a functioning renal allograft for 20 years or longer, all enjoyed excellent and stable renal function; their mean serum creatinine level at 20 years was 1.3 mg/dL. On the other hand, eight patients experienced complications related to long-term immunosuppressive therapy and infection; seven, malignancy; and six, cardiovascular disease.[66a]

Psychologic Adaptation to Transplantation

The immediate postoperative psychologic status of the patient can vary enormously. The patient realizes that his or her fate hangs on the daily blood analyses. Even if the uremia is improving, long-term complications may develop. In the case of a cadaver recipient, there may be feelings of an "anticlimax" following the enormous excitement of being called after waiting a long time for a kidney to become available.

If the patient has been on dialysis, his or her lifestyle and family structure have been altered. Adjustments will now be necessary from life on dialysis to life with a transplant. Many patients imagine that all their problems will disappear after the transplant. They need to be counseled that transplantation is not a "cure" for their disease—it is another mode of therapy. They must be aware of the complications listed earlier, but they also need to know that their quality of life will most likely improve.

Nursing Management

The postoperative nursing management for the *donor* is the same as that following a nephrectomy (discussed later). The *recipient* needs the usual postoperative nursing management, plus close observation of the urinary output and monitoring of creatinine and potassium laboratory values, and protective measures to prevent infection because of immunosuppression.

Discharge Planning and Community Care: Posttransplant

Major points to stress in the posttransplant teaching follow.

- *Administer medications correctly.* Because medications have a large role in the treatment and must be taken for life, it is important that the patient take them accurately.
- *Restrict activity for 2 to 3 months following surgery.* The recipient kidney placed close to the surface in the iliac fossa must be protected. Advise the patient to resume pretransplant activity level slowly and steadily; swimming and bicycle riding are good forms of exercise.
- *Weigh daily; take temperature and blood pressure twice daily; measure urine output, and record on daily record sheet.* This information is essential in recognizing a rejection episode.
- *Report signs of rejection to the physician immediately:* fever, swelling and tenderness of the graft site, decreased urinary output, respiratory distress, increasing blood pressure, weight gain, blood in the urine, and general weakness. The earlier the rejection is recognized and treated, the better are the chances of reversing it.
- *Avoid strong sunlight by protecting the skin from exposure.* The incidence of skin cancer in patients taking immunosuppressive drugs is higher than in the general population. Other cancers may also develop.
- *If appropriate, discuss family planning.* After a transplant, sexual function may be restored. Pregnancy has a minimal adverse effect on kidney function.
- *Look for signs of infection. Avoid large groups of people for about 3 months postoperatively.* Immunosuppressive drugs increase susceptibility to infection. Instruct the patient to contact the physician if there is any sign of infection in any form.
- *Comply with diet restrictions.* They may be necessary to help maintain blood pressure, body weight, and blood values within normal limits. Sodium, potassium, fluids, and calories will be modified individually.

Community care is especially important. All patients are prescribed antirejection agents. Sudden discontinuance of these drugs can cause a severe rejection episode. Immunologic follow-up is done to permit early detection of rejection and to adjust immunosuppressive therapy, allowing the optimum dose rather than the maximum tolerated dose to be prescribed. The patient is also observed for early signs of the complications listed earlier so that early treatment may be instituted.

Evaluation/Desired Outcomes. The patient with a renal transplant will:

1. Maintain satisfactory fluid, electrolyte, and acid–base balance
2. Experience no complications related to surgery and medication therapy
3. Experience a satisfactory psychosocial adjustment and achieve as near normal a lifestyle as possible
4. Be able to verbalize and implement pertinent information related to diet and medication therapies
5. Keep follow-up appointments
6. Be able to verbalize the signs and symptoms of complications, including rejection, which should be reported to the physician

■ THE KIDNEYS AND SYSTEMIC DISORDERS

Systemic disorders may cause structural and functional alterations of the kidney. The renal injury is secondary to another disease process, so the prescribed care is often more complicated. Two major types of systemic disorders causing nephropathy, diabetes mellitus and hypertension, are discussed, as are less common disorders causing nephropathy.

Diabetic Nephropathy

Patients who have had diabetes mellitus for a variable number of years are likely to develop complications that include retinopathy, neuropathy, and nephropathy. Diabetics are also more prone than the normal population to develop urinary tract infection and chronic pyelonephritis. Diabetic nephropathy is a complex disorder thought to result primarily from an alteration in glomerular capillaries.

It has been estimated that 30% of the population in the United States with ESRD have renal disease related to diabetes mellitus. Diabetic nephropathy may be due to both genetic factors and metabolic alterations that vary among patients. Approximately 50 to 60% of the patients have insulin-dependent diabetes mellitus (IDDM).

The glomerular changes are not present early in the disorder but can be detected after several years.[34] There is extensive diffuse glomerular and arteriolar involvement. The glomeruli gradually lose their fine structure and become replaced by shapeless masses of tissue that can no longer act as filters; thus proteinuria results. The major renal arteries and their branches are arteriosclerotic in most patients with diabetes, thereby contributing to hypertension and reducing renal blood flow. In advanced nephropathy, tubular atrophy occurs. The *Kimmelsteil–Wilson lesion* is the histologic finding specific to diabetes. Of patients who develop diabetic nephropathy, most do so within 10 to 30 years of the onset of the diabetes.

Five classic *clinical findings* of diabetic nephropathy are proteinuria, hypertension, azotemia, edema, and recurrent urinary tract infections with papillary necrosis. Proteinuria, occasionally in the nephrotic range, is the clinical hallmark of diabetic nephropathy; edema may be massive. Renal function usually deteriorates gradually. Once azotemia develops, ESRD will soon follow. As the urinary output decreases, urine tests for glucose and acetone lose their value, because urine glucose levels no longer reflect serum glucose levels.

No specific *treatment* has yet been discovered to influence the renal lesion caused by diabetes, but renal disease may be minimized or postponed with careful control of diabetes mellitus (discussed in Chap. 46), treatment of infection, and management of hypertension. A low protein diet and treatment with an angiotensin converting enzyme inhibitor (ACE) may also be helpful. When azotemia develops, the outlook is poor. Death from renal or vascular disease will occur unless dialysis or transplantation is initiated.

Dietary problems increase as renal failure advances, because the nutritional management of diabetes conflicts with that of renal disease. Adequate protein intake is needed in the diabetic diet, but protein intake needs to be restricted in the renal failure diet to lessen the work of the kidneys when the patient is being treated conservatively.

Insulin needs usually drop drastically as renal function deteriorates. In addition, the diabetic is generally encouraged to maintain an adequate fluid intake, yet the fluids have to be restricted when there is an inadequate urinary output. Thirst from hyperglycemia will be difficult to handle for the diabetic with a compromised urinary output.

Hypertension and Nephrosclerosis

Two types of hypertension associated with renal pathology are benign essential hypertension and malignant hypertension. Both types affect the small arteries and arterioles of the kidneys. A major determinant of the type and severity of the renal involvement appears to be the severity of the hypertension.[34] These renal abnormalities are referred to as *benign arteriolar nephrosclerosis* and *malignant arteriolar nephrosclerosis*.

It is estimated that one in four adults in the United States has high blood pressure. Hypertension is the second leading cause of CRF in the United States, probably resulting from inadequate treatment, patient noncompliance, or delayed diagnosis of hypertension.

In benign nephrosclerosis, on microscopic examination of the arterioles, there is marked thickening and necrosis of the walls, reduced size of the lumen, fibrin deposits, and tubular atrophy. The kidneys in malignant nephrosclerosis vary in size from normal to moderately contracted. Petechial hemorrhages are commonly found on the surface of the kidneys and at times are extremely diffuse and prominent. Renal blood flow and the glomerular filtration rate may be greatly reduced. The damaged kidneys cannot perform their usual regulation of the amount of sodium and water retained in the body, and so this altered function further aggravates the hypertension because of volume expansion.

In *essential hypertension,* renal failure progresses if the blood pressure is not controlled. In *malignant hypertension,* the diastolic blood pressure is frequently greater than

130 mm Hg, and protein and blood are present in the urine. Urinalyses may reveal hyaline and granular casts, RBCs, WBCs, proteinuria, and albuminuria. If the blood pressure is not controlled, creatinine clearance studies show progressive reduction of renal function. Renal failure rapidly occurs if the blood pressure is not lowered. The major goal of treatment is reduction of the blood pressure.

Less Common Systemic Disorders Causing Nephropathy

Renovascular Hypertension. Renovascular hypertension is caused by stenosis of one or both renal arteries from atherosclerotic plaques, abnormal tissue in the vessels, or occlusion of the renal artery with emboli, leading to ischemia of the kidney. The *clinical findings* are similar to those of any patient with essential hypertension, but should be specifically ruled out in patients (1) with abrupt onset, (2) under 20 or over 50 years of age, and (3) with no history of hypertension in the family. A renal arteriogram may be necessary for diagnosis. The *treatment* is medical intervention with antihypertensives or reconstructive surgery if needed, such as an aortorenal bypass graft or renal angioplasty.

Lupus Glomerulonephritis. Systemic lupus erythematosus (SLE) can lead to glomerulonephritis by producing an immunologic injury to the glomeruli that ranges from minimal glomerular alterations to diffuse, proliferative involvement. The clinical features of renal involvement have little relationship to the severity of the glomerular lesions. *Clinical findings* include proteinuria, which may lead to the nephrotic syndrome. There is an increase in urinary sediment, including RBC, WBC, and hyaline casts. Hypertension and renal failure may develop. The *treatment* includes steroids, plasmapheresis, and/or cytotoxic drugs. Some patients develop progressive renal disease and require dialysis.

Amyloidosis. Amyloidosis is the deposit in the glomerulus of amyloid, a proteinlike material with a waxy texture that replaces the normal cells. These deposits also tend to localize within blood vessels and tissues of the liver, spleen, heart, and GI tract. The disease can be primary, with no apparent cause, or secondary to some other disease process.

Clinical findings commonly include proteinuria in the nephrotic range and enlarged kidneys. Hypertension is frequently absent. A rectal biopsy normally confirms the diagnosis; amyloid deposits are more accessible in this area than in the kidney and the procedure is less dangerous than a kidney biopsy. There is no satisfactory *treatment* for amyloidosis. Dialysis is performed for renal failure. The prognosis is poor once the nephrotic syndrome and azotemia develop.

Goodpasture's Syndrome. Goodpasture's syndrome is a severe form of acute glomerulonephritis that frequently leads to progressive renal damage. Antibodies develop against the glomeruli that may also act against the alveoli in the lungs. This condition occurs primarily in young males between 20 and 30 years of age. *Clinical findings* include mild to moderate proteinuria, recurrent pulmonary hemorrhages leading to hemoptysis, and dyspnea of varying degrees. An upper respiratory infection may precede the onset. Early *treatment* by plasmapheresis may remove the offending antibody, saving the kidneys and lungs from further damage. Treatment of the renal failure is dialysis. Steroids and cytotoxic drugs may be administered. Long periods of remission from pulmonary hemorrhage may occur.

Polyarteritis Nodosa. Polyarteritis nodosa is a form of systemic vasculitis (inflammation of blood vessels). In the kidney, there is acute inflammation of medium-size (arcuate and interlobar) blood vessels. *Clinical findings* include hematuria and hypertension. There may be infarction of the kidneys. Progressive renal failure is a late manifestation. Vigorous *treatment* of the hypertension is important. Steroids may be administered.

Sickle Cell Nephropathy. Sickle cell nephropathy results from occlusion of small vessels by RBCs. The capillary beds enlarge and the capillaries contain sickled RBCs. Cortical infarctions and papillary necrosis develop. The *clinical findings* are those of sickle cell disease. The most common finding is painless gross hematuria. Proteinuria is usual, but the nephrotic syndrome is uncommon. Hypertension is not a consistent finding. *Treatment* in the end stage is chronic dialysis.

■ RENAL INFECTIONS

Types of renal infections include pyelonephritis and renal tuberculosis.

Pyelonephritis

The term *pyelonephritis* actually refers to inflammation of the kidney and its pelvis, but more commonly connotes bacterial infection of the kidney tissue (parenchyma) and the renal pelvis, as in *acute pyelonephritis*. It is now thought that a variety of nonbacterial infections and chemical, physical, and immunologic factors can also produce the tubulointerstitial changes that occur with *chronic pyelonephritis*. In addition, in the majority of cases of chronic pyelonephritis, the infection is superimposed on an anatomic urinary tract anomaly, a urinary obstruction, or vesicoureteral reflux (condition that allows infected urine from the bladder to ascend to the kidney).[34]

The infection usually begins in the lower urinary tract, ascending the mucosa of the urethra, bladder, and ureter to the kidney pelvis, and then to the parenchyma. The role of bacterial adherence to the mucosa is being studied as a predisposing factor.[34] Occasionally an infection can be carried in the blood (called a *hematogenous infection*) to the kidneys. Lower urinary tract infection may be asymptomatic, with the kidney involvement being the first sign of a lower urinary tract disorder.

Over 85% of urinary infections are caused by bacterial species that normally inhabit the intestinal tract, such as *Escherichia coli, Proteus,* and *Klebsiella. E. coli* is the most common organism identified in pyelonephritis, and resistance to antibiotic therapy rarely occurs.[10]

Incidence and Epidemiology. Urinary tract infection is one of the most common of all bacterial disorders. Infections range in severity from simple bacterial growth in the urine without symptoms to massive renal infection resulting in chronic renal failure. When urinary tract infections are superimposed on anatomic abnormalities, calculous disease, or analgesic abuse, they appear to have an important role in the development of chronic renal disease.[34]

There is a marked preponderance of pyelonephritis in females, with contributing factors being urethral trauma during intercourse and a short urethra. Enlarged prostates in males may obstruct urine flow, which can also lead to pyelonephritis. Pyelonephritis may be associated with instrumentation (i.e., catheterization, cystoscopy, and urologic surgery) and chronic health problems.

Autopsy studies have revealed a high incidence of chronic pyelonephritis in diabetics.[34] Increased urinary glucose concentration, a tendency to obesity, neuropathy, and angiopathy have all been suggested as causative factors. Persons with various forms of glomerular, tubular, and vascular renal disorders also have been reported to show an increased frequency of pyelonephritis.

The normal bladder, kidneys, and urine are sterile; however, urine is a reasonably good culture medium for organisms that cause urinary tract infections (UTIs). Vesicoureteral reflux and intrarenal reflux (spread of infection from the pelvis of the kidney through open ducts of the papillae into the cortex) are two main pathologic factors contributing to the progression of ascending infection from the bladder to the kidney.

Nursing Management: Prevention and Reduction of Risk Factors. Nurses can aid in the prevention of pyelonephritis in the following ways:

1. Teach the female patient to wipe the perineal area from front to back after voiding or defecating. This prevents contamination of the urethral area by organisms of the GI tract found in feces or in secretions from the vagina. Females should also urinate after sexual intercourse.

2. In the catheterized patient, provide periurethral care, maintain the closed drainage system, and position the tubing and bag so that flow of urine is unobstructed.

3. Teach patients requiring chronic urinary drainage about the importance of (1) handwashing before and after catheter care, (2) the long-term antimicrobial regimen that may be prescribed, (3) the correct procedure for bladder irrigations, and (4) an adequate fluid intake (at least 3 L daily in the absence of cardiovascular problems).

4. Stress the importance of wearing gloves and of meticulous handwashing for all personnel who are responsible for intravenous care to assist in preventing the hematogenous spread of infection to the kidneys.

5. Participate in mass screening to identify asymptomatic persons who need treatment for pyelonephritis, thus assisting in decreasing the long-term complications of hypertension and renal failure.

Pathophysiology, Clinical Findings, Diagnostic Studies, Treatment, Complications, and Prognosis. Clinically pyelonephritis may be acute or chronic, symptomatic or asymptomatic. The severity of the symptoms is not related to the severity of the disease. Table 48–16 compares acute and chronic pyelonephritis. Figure 48–7 shows the progressive changes in the kidney from pyelonephritis.

Pyelonephritis in the elderly may cause an acute confused state with incontinence or a general deterioration of the physical condition and behavior. Urinalysis and culture and sensitivity of the urine will confirm the diagnosis.

Nursing Management. The goal of nursing management is to teach the patient ways to reduce and control the bacterial population of the urinary tract to prevent or retard the progression of renal damage. Nursing management includes the nursing measures related to the therapies. It is especially important to encourage fluid intake. Cranberry juice, which acidifies the urine, can also be used.[5]

TABLE 48–16

COMPARISON OF ACUTE AND CHRONIC PYELONEPHRITIS

	Acute Pyelonephritis (APN)	Chronic Pyelonephritis (CPN)
Pathophysiology	Severity varies from simple pyelitis (infecting pelvic mucosa) to involvement of entire lobes of the medulla and cortex. Kidneys with severe APN are enlarged and contain abscesses. Calices enlarge and become obstructed. Interstitium is edematous; tubules are necrotic. All renal structures (glomeruli, blood vessels, and tubules) within abscesses are destroyed, but this is localized and not diffuse.	Renal pelvis and calices are continuously inflamed. As acute renal parenchymal inflammation subsides, fibrous tissue may replace damaged structures and form a scar; there is a visible shrinkage of kidney tissue in this area. Coexisting infection is usually present. Presence of hypertension will lead to renal arteriolar disease, which contributes to more extensive renal disease.
Clinical findings	High fever, backache, abdominal pain or tenderness, chills, costovertebral angle (CVA) tenderness over the involved side, headache, malaise, anorexia are major findings. Hypotension is present in severe cases. Clinical findings persist for one to several days. Urine may be cloudy with an ammonia odor.	Hypertension is major finding. Clear-cut symptoms of infection may be entirely lacking despite presence of bacteria in urine, or renal colic may be first sign. Vague flank or abdominal pain, intermittent low-grade fever, and symptoms of lower urinary tract infection may be present. Polyuria and nocturia may occur early in the course.
Diagnostic studies	Urinalysis reveals pyuria, hematuria, clumps of bacteria, WBC casts, and minimal proteinuria. Leukocytosis is present. In uncomplicated cases, renal function is normal (BUN is normal). In severe obstruction or infection, azotemia is present.	*Radiologic findings:* Excretory urogram, voiding cystourethrography, postvoiding cystograms, cystoscopy, and gynecologic evaluation may detect presence of vesicoureteral reflux or obstruction. *Urinalysis:* Bacteriuria may be present but urine is often sterile. Pyuria may be present. Proteinuria is infrequent unless hypertension or renal insufficiency is present.
Treatment	Antibiotic therapy may be parenteral initially if severe illness is present, then orally. Antipyretics are given to control fever. Adequate fluid intake is 3 L daily unless contraindicated. Structural defects, such as vesicoureteral reflux or urinary obstruction from a renal calculus, are surgically corrected.	Antihypertensive therapy is given and adequate fluid intake (3 L daily unless contraindicated) encouraged. Repeated infections will require routine laboratory work and reexamination periodically.
Complications	Septicemia	Renal failure
Prognosis	Usual course without complications following *Escherichia coli* infection is healing rather than progressive damage. Phase of acute inflammation in kidney lasts from 1 to 3 weeks. By the 6th to 10th week kidneys are sterile with a resultant scar. *Staphyloccocus, Klebsiella,* and *Streptococcus faecalis* infections tend to persist longer.	With persistent inflammation, the disease takes a progressive downward course.

(Source: *Jacobson and Striker.*[34])

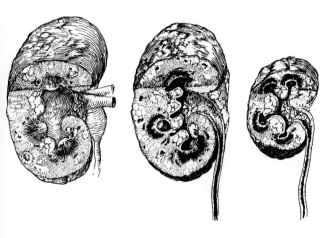

Figure 48–7. Progressive pathologic changes in kidney resulting from re-peated attacks of acute pyelonephritis with progressive scarring. **Left:** Early stage of focal parenchymal scarring. **Center:** Progressive scarring with nar-rowing of necks of calices, causing caliceal dilation. **Right:** End stage of re-current pyelonephritis (stage of atrophy) (*From Tanagho and McAninch.*[79])

Discharge Planning and Community Care

Discharge planning should incorporate teaching about the following:

1. The importance of an adequate fluid intake (at least 3 L/day in the absence of cardiovascular problems)

2. The importance of taking prescribed antibiotics to treat the infection

3. The nature of the disorder and how the antibiotics can help to prevent permanent kidney damage

4. The importance of complying with the request to have urine cultures repeated periodically so that the status of the urinary system can be evaluated and recurrent episodes of infection can be identified

5. The signs and symptoms of kidney infection and the need to seek health care without delay

During community visits the patient should be asked about symptoms of dysuria, cloudy urine, frequent small voidings, fever, pain, and headaches. Some antibiotics are extremely expensive; the patient can be asked discreetly about the financial status and if the prescribed medications have been obtained. Refer the patient to a social worker if financial problems are identified. Emergency funds are sometimes available from community agencies for such needs. Some drug companies provide reduced rates to those persons in need.

Evaluation/Desired Outcomes. The patient will:

1. Understand and comply with antibiotic therapy

2. Return for follow-up urine cultures as instructed

3. Be able to verbalize signs and symptoms that should be reported promptly (dysuria, flank pain, suprapubic pain, nausea, and vomiting)

4. If infection is persistent, return for regular visits for fol-low-up and blood pressure control if indicated

Renal Tuberculosis

Renal tuberculosis (TB or TBC) is a special form of urinary tract infection that may or may not accompany pulmonary tuberculosis and may remain asymptomatic for years while irreversible renal destruction takes place. Pulmonary TB is discussed in Chap. 35. This section will highlight only renal TB. *Mycobacterium tuberculosis* is the causative organism. Of the new cases of TB reported annually, approximately 15% are extrapulmonary, with the genitourinary tract as the leading site.[34]

The tubercle bacilli are hematogenously carried throughout the body and may lodge in the kidneys. The dis-ease involves the renal cortex and/or medulla with tissue destruction in all directions. The renal lesion is usually nodular and fibrotic with severe scarring; calcifications with irregular cavities may appear as the disease progresses. Once the infection reaches the pelvis, it moves down the urinary tract and involves other urinary tissue. Fibrosis and stenosis of the ureter caused by the organism may prevent pus and urine from leaving the infected kidney, which ac-celerates renal destruction.

Symptoms of pulmonary TB may precede renal symp-toms. Weight loss, general malaise, low-grade fever, dysuria, hematuria, flank pain, and pyuria are the most frequent pre-senting *clinical findings* for active urinary TB; however, the disease often produces only vague symptoms. Symptoms secondary to tuberculous infection of the kidney that involve the male urinary and reproductive tract affect the prostate, seminal vesicles, vas deferens, epididymis, and testes.

A positive skin test is present in most patients with renal TB. Excretory urograms show a "moth-eaten" appearance of the calices with evidence of calcification as the disease pro-gresses. Excretion of the bacilli into the urine is intermittent, which may cause a negative urine culture. Multiple (up to 12) urine cultures are suggested before renal TB is ruled out. The specimens are usually collected on successive mornings with the first voided specimen being the most accurate.

Treatment is with antituberculosis drugs. Corticoste-roids may be used to reduce scarring. Chemotherapy is highly effective; partial or total nephrectomy may be neces-sary if there is persistent infection that does not respond to chemotherapy. Permanent urinary diversion or reconstruc-tive ureteral surgery may be necessary with severe strictures or irreparable bladder damage.

Nursing management is discussed in Chap. 35. In the collection of urine specimens, special precautions should be taken when handling the urine because it is presumed to be infectious. Gloves should be worn and the specimen should be labeled as possibly infectious. It is not necessary to wear a mask. Any urine or urinary bags should be isolated and disposed of correctly. The urine should be observed for evi-dence of hematuria and pyuria.

■ ADULT POLYCYSTIC KIDNEY DISEASE

In polycystic kidney disease (PKD) of adults, cysts develop throughout the cortex and medulla (Fig. 48–8). PKD is the most common renal cystic disorder in adults, excluding the simple renal cyst. Approximately 5% of patients on dialysis in the United States have PKD.[82] It affects the sexes equally and has a similar course in both sexes. Most patients are initially diagnosed between 35 and 45 years. The average age at the time of death or initiation of dialysis is between 50 and 57 years.

PKD is transmitted primarily as an autosomal dominant trait. A family history of PKD can be obtained in 50 to 70%; 100% of gene carriers develop the disease by the age of 80, but this does not mean that all patients with PKD will progress to uremia.[34]

Adult PKD is a structural disorder of both kidneys in which cysts of varying size occupy or displace much of the renal parenchyma, resulting in enlargement as much as 10 times normal volume, thus displacing other abdominal organs. Individual cysts vary from less than 1 mm to more than 5 cm in diameter. In about one third of patients, cysts also occur in the liver, but they generally do not interfere with liver function. Cysts may also occur in the pancreas, spleen, thyroid, and gonads. These patients also have a higher incidence of intracranial aneurysms. PKD is a slowly progressive condition, and so it is often initially asymptomatic.[34] Renal calculi are common in these patients. When sudden or unexplained deterioration in renal function occurs, obstruction from renal calculi may be the cause.

Clinical Findings

The cardinal feature of PKD is palpable bilateral abdominal masses. Kidney size corresponds fairly well with renal function; if the kidneys are not palpable on physical examination, renal function may be normal. There is a marked reduction in ability to concentrate urine, as evidenced by

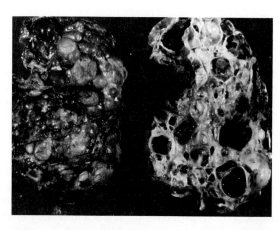

Figure 48–8. Adult polycystic disease of the kidneys. One kidney has been bisected to show both external (**left**) and internal (**right**) surfaces. Note multiple cysts with loss of renal substance. (*From Chandrosoma and Taylor.*[14])

polyuria and nocturia. Dysuria may or may not be present. Hypertension is very common and may precede impairment of renal function. Lumbar, flank, or abdominal pain is a common presenting symptom.[34] The specific causes for pain are multiple, including ureteral obstruction related to calculi, infection, spontaneous hemorrhage into a cyst, or a ruptured cyst.

Diagnostic Studies

Microscopic or macroscopic hematuria; pyuria, which suggests rupture of a cyst; and moderate proteinuria are frequently present. Pyelonephritis is common and may accelerate the rate of deterioration of renal function. Cystic disease is confirmed with magnetic resonance imaging (MRI), an excretory urogram, ultrasound, nephrotomogram, or arteriography.

Even at low levels of renal function, anemia is frequently absent because kidney size is increased and erythropoietin production is not decreased. *Erythrocytosis* (hematocrit over 60%) has been reported, even with azotemia. The rate at which the glomerular filtration rate decreases with progression of the disease is slow when compared to other renal diseases.

Treatment

The goals of treatment of PKD are to normalize the blood pressure, prevent or treat urinary tract infection or obstruction, and manage renal pain. A diuretic and salt restriction are initial treatments. The addition of an antihypertensive is usually sufficient to control the blood pressure in most patients. Careful assessments are of utmost importance in determining the need for further treatment and evaluating the effect of the current regimen.

Recurrent or chronic lumbar, flank, or abdominal pain—a feeling of uncomfortable "heaviness" in the abdomen resulting from enlargement of the kidneys—is part of the usual course of the disease. Addictive and nephrotoxic analgesics should be avoided. If the pain is severe, calculi should be ruled out.

Massive hematuria may become a problem with renal calculi, so the urine should be closely observed. While surgical decompression of cysts provides no beneficial long-term effects on the glomerular filtration, surgery may be indicated if there is obstruction of the urinary tract by the cysts.

Management of CRF resulting from PKD includes successful hemodialysis and renal transplantation. Survival of the patient and graft in transplantation is not less in PKD than in other forms of ESRD. The presence of PKD is an important factor in advising these patients in regard to the possibility that the condition will be transmitted to their children.

Complications and Prognosis

The most devastating extrarenal complication associated with PKD is congenital aneurysm of the cerebral arteries. Any patient with PKD who complains of a headache or develops any neurologic signs should undergo careful diagnostic evaluation for a cerebral aneurysm.[34] Any of these findings should be reported to the physician.

In spite of the long course of this disease, patients with PKD and chronic renal failure often appear relatively well despite the presence of azotemia; this is partially due to the absence of anemia. The presence of hypertension and its control are major determinants of the prognosis of PKD.

Nursing Management

Family and individual counseling are important. Ultrasound is the preferred method to screen family members. The need for continuing care after hospitalization cannot be overemphasized. The patient should notify his or her health care professional when there are any signs of infection, increased hematuria, or unusual pain.

■ RENAL OBSTRUCTIVE DISEASE

Obstruction can be unilateral or bilateral, painless or painful, with or without infection; the clinical situation is much more severe if infection is present. Acute urinary tract obstruction often causes obvious clinical symptoms, whereas chronic obstruction is often asymptomatic. Table 48–17 lists some common causes of urinary obstruction and where they may occur in the urinary tract.

Obstruction of the urinary tract at any level is a common cause of acute or chronic renal failure. When recognized, it is usually treatable by surgical measures, and renal failure is often prevented or reversed.

HYDRONEPHROSIS

Hydronephrosis refers to a dilation of the collecting system of the kidney (renal pelvis and calices) and the structural changes in the kidney caused by an obstruction to the flow of urine.

Incidence and Epidemiology

The incidence of hydronephrosis at autopsy is about 4%. The clinical frequency of obstruction is lower, but it is a rather common problem.[10] During the middle years, hydronephrosis is more common in women than in men because of the frequency of pregnancy and cancer of the pelvic organs. In the young adult male, calculous disease is the most common cause of acute hydronephrosis. Later in life, men with hydronephrosis outnumber women as a result of benign and malignant prostatic disease and urethral strictures.

Pathophysiology

Figure 48–9 illustrates the pathologic changes associated with obstruction and the resultant hydronephrosis. Normal mechanisms of urine formation depend on the progressive decrease in hydrostatic pressure from the renal artery to the bladder, so changes in this pressure can affect renal function. There is no actual primary pathology of the nephron,

TABLE 48–17

COMMON CAUSES OF URINARY OBSTRUCTION

Level of Obstruction	Pathologic Obstruction
All levels	Calculi[a,b] Trauma Blood clots Papillary tissue
Tubule	Uric acid crystals Polycystic kidneys (from cysts)
Renal pelvis	Ectopic kidney Tuberculosis Fibrous bands or stricture at the ureteropelvic junction
Ureter	Abdominal and pelvic neoplasms[b] Lymphoma and metastatic cancer Retroperitoneal fibrosis or abscess Stricture Diverticulum Endometriosis Pregnancy[a]
Bladder	Benign prostatic hypertrophy[b] Foreign body Contraction of bladder neck Cancer of the prostate[b] Cancer of the bladder Neurogenic bladder[b] Prostatic abscesses
Urethra	Diverticulum Meatal stenosis Stricture (congenital or acquired from infection or trauma)[b] Foreign body Cancer of urethra or penis Ectopic ureter

[a]Most prevalent causes of obstruction of urinary tract in adult female.
[b]Most prevalent causes of obstruction of urinary tract in adult male.
(Source: *Brenner and Rector.*[10])

so urine production continues, and then the urine is trapped proximal to the obstruction. Continuous urine production increases the volume and intrapelvic pressure in the passageway, which can lead to nephron destruction and renal failure.

Clinical Findings

A thorough history needs to be obtained from the patient with obstructive disease, inquiring about malignancy, previous surgery, pain, hematuria, and fever. The female is asked about endometriosis and pelvic inflammatory disease.

When obstruction occurs in the ureter or kidney, the patient complains of pain in the flank radiating along the

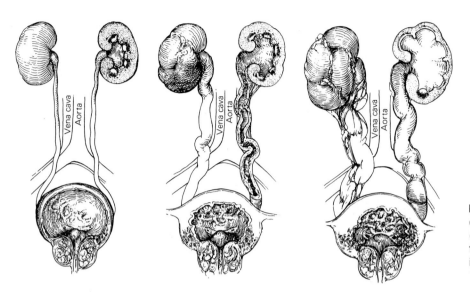

Figure 48–9. Pathogenesis of bilateral hydronephrosis. Progressive changes in bladder (thickened wall), ureters (dilation and elongation), and kidneys (dilation of pelves and calices) are caused by enlarged prostate. (*From Tanagho and McAninch.*[79])

course of the ureter. Infection causes chills, fever, and burning on urination.[79]

Diagnostic Studies

The urinalysis, urine culture, CBC, and serum creatinine will be monitored. The urinalysis may be normal, but RBCs and WBCs are usually present. Proteinuria is absent or mild in most cases. In obstructive disease with slowing of intratubular fluid flow, there may be increased reabsorption of urea in the distal nephron. Thus, the BUN may be elevated out of proportion to the serum creatinine, the ratio normally being 10:1. Serial measurements of creatinine clearance may be required for assessment of renal function.

Radiologic evaluation such as an excretory urogram may be difficult because of obstruction to the flow of urine in the urinary system and to the contrast medium in the circulatory system. Contrast medium is often seen puddling in the hydronephrotic renal pelvis because of the reduced glomerular filtration rate resulting from obstruction of blood flow, and it may accumulate in the renal cortex. The contrast medium enters the parenchyma eventually and delayed films (up to 24 to 36 hours) usually demonstrate the level of obstruction.

Treatment

The goals for treatment of hydronephrosis are to relieve the obstruction, prevent volume depletion and electrolyte imbalances caused by postobstructive diuresis, preserve renal function, and prevent infection. Emergency surgical relief of the obstruction may be necessary. Removal of the obstruction causes a sudden decrease in the pressure on the renal parenchyma exerted by the trapped urine. This leads to a temporary postobstructive diuresis that can persist for a few hours or a few days. It can cause fluid depletion and shock if the patient is not monitored closely and fluid is not adequately replaced.

Complications and Prognosis

Complications of hydronephrosis include renal failure, pyelonephritis, hypertension, polycythemia, and lithiasis. The development of *renal failure* may require immediate treatment by dialysis until the obstruction can be corrected. There is increased risk of *pyelonephritis* because of urinary stasis, reflux, and suboptimal urinary drainage. Gram-negative septicemia may occur if pyelonephritis develops in the presence of obstruction.

Hypertension is associated with chronic hydronephrosis. Bilateral hydronephrosis results in sodium retention and volume expansion, which can lead to volume-dependent hypertension. Acute obstruction may cause renin to be released, thus elevating systemic blood pressure.

Polycythemia, an unusual complication of hydronephrosis, appears to be secondary to increased erythropoietin secretion by the obstructed kidney.[10] The infected hydronephrotic kidney is prone to formation of struvite *stones.* Once the triad of infection, obstruction, and urolithiasis is present, it is difficult to eliminate. The prognosis depends on the chronicity of the condition.

Nursing Management

During the obstructive phase, nursing management is directed toward providing for the patient's comfort and relief of pain, plus monitoring the urinary output, blood pressure, fluid status, and serum and urinary laboratory tests.

When the patient is unable to void, the physician may request a catheterized specimen. The catheter should be lubricated well before placement and passed very gently without force. If obstruction is met, the physician should be notified; a suprapubic catheter may be inserted. After the patient is able to void, the volume of residual urine may be measured.

After the obstruction is removed, the patient's urine output, specific gravity, and vital signs are carefully monitored. Fluid management during this period is a priority. Hourly fluid replacement is usually based on the amount of the previous hour's urinary output. Periodic serum electrolyte and glucose levels are done, and any significant changes are reported to the physician immediately. A low serum sodium (less than 135) should be especially noted, because this electrolyte may be lost in large quantities.

The patient may be weak from excess urinary losses. Rest should be promoted by encouraging frequent quiet periods and comfortable positioning while in bed, by limiting visitation, and by having a calm, quiet approach. The prescribed antibiotics are administered and the patient is assessed for signs of infection. *Discharge planning* and *community care* are related to the cause of the hydronephrosis, discussed in the section on Epidemiology.

RENAL CALCULI

Renal stones (calculi) begin developing on the surfaces of the papillae and are an example of soft tissue calcification. When stones become detached, they accompany urine as it flows into the collecting system. They are often too large to pass through the renal pelvis, ureters, or urethra. Therefore, they may obstruct the flow of urine, causing severe pain and hydronephrosis.

Incidence and Epidemiology

Renal calculi affect up to 5% of the population, with a recurrence rate in afflicted individuals of 50 to 80%.[10]

Patients who have *gout* may form uric acid stones. Many patients who form *calcium stones* have increased urinary excretion of calcium. The presence of urinary tract infection is a nidus (point of origin) in the formation of struvite stones, which can increase in size and fill the renal pelvis and calices. They are called *staghorn calculi* (Fig. 48–10). If urinary stasis and hydronephrosis are also present, the chances of calculus formation are increased. Conversely, a calculus may produce obstruction and urinary stasis, which predispose to infection. Not all persons with the aforementioned conditions form stones.

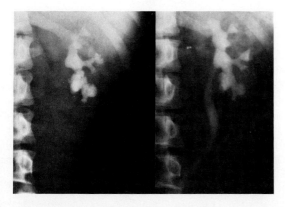

Figure 48–10. Staghorn stone. **Left:** KUB. **Right:** IVP. (*From Tanagho and McAninch.*[79])

Geographic "stone belts" have been described in areas in the world where the incidence of urinary calculi is high. Calcium oxalate stones are the most common stones in North America. Hot climates also favor stone formation. If fluid intake is not adequate, urinary output decreases and the urine becomes more concentrated, so that precipitation of dissolved salts is more likely.

Nursing Management: Prevention and Reduction of Risk Factors

Nurses can assist in teaching about the prevention of stones in the following ways:

1. Teach the patient the importance of adequate, consistent fluid intake to prevent stone formation. Whatever the basic pathologic condition that leads to the formation of stones, a high urine volume will dilute any substances that may be precipitated and will decrease calculus formation. Advise the patient to drink one glass of fluid every hour while awake during the day. Although a high fluid intake is necessary to produce a high urine volume, it is more practical to emphasize the need for a high urine volume because it is more convenient for the patient to measure urine output than fluid intake. A high urine volume means at least 2 L, or possibly up to 3 or 4 L, per 24 hours. If the patient has diarrhea or diaphoresis, fluid intake should be increased to compensate for the excessive losses. If the fluid depletion is caused by vomiting, it may be necessary to maintain fluid intake intravenously.

2. Because the incidence of stone disease among the families of stone formers is much higher than in the general population, teach the patient's family the clinical signs of stone disease so that they can identify and immediately report any symptoms to their health care professional and seek proper treatment.

3. Teach the patient the importance of identifying and reporting symptoms of urinary tract infections promptly to prevent further stress on the kidneys.

Pathophysiology

Urinary stones are formed by the following general principles, regardless of the specific type of calculus: *Crystalluria* (excess crystals in the urine) leads to *nucleation* (spontaneous formation of new crystals in an oversaturated solution) and ultimately to *new crystal* (calculus) *growth.* Calculi will continue to enlarge in oversaturated urine.

The multiple types of renal stones may be composed of one substance or mixtures of several materials. Table 48–18 lists information concerning five different types of stones listed according to frequency of occurrence.

Clinical Findings

All types of stones present with virtually the same clinical findings as the result of obstruction and tissue trauma. Points of anatomic ureteral narrowing include the uteropelvic junction, about midpoint where the ureter crosses the iliac vessels, and the ureterovesical junction. The position of the stone determines the clinical findings. An obstructing

TABLE 48–18

RENAL STONES RELATIVE TO FREQUENCY OF OCCURRENCE

Calcium Stones

Incidence	Calcium stones are the most common type in North America; 80% of all urinary tract stones contain calcium. Highest incidence is at 30 to 50 years of age, and it occurs three times more often in men than women.
Special clinical problems	Recurrence is the rule; 11% of calcium stone formers produce very large numbers of stones. Risk of calcium stone formation increases with hypercalciuria, oxaluria, alkaline urine, and dehydration. Hypercalciuria results from (1) hyperparathyroidism, (2) increased calcium absorption from GI tract, and (3) impaired renal tubular absorption of filtered calcium.
Dietary intervention	Restrict all dairy products. Avoid vitamin D–enriched foods. Increase fluid intake to maintain urinary output of 2 L or more daily.
Medications	
Cellulose phosphate	Calcium binding resin that decreases intestinal absorption of calcium.
Hydrochlorothiazide	Increases renal tubular reabsorption of calcium, which decreases oxalate saturation and prevents some stone formation.

Oxalate Stones

Incidence	Oxalate stones are most common in areas where cereals and vegetables are major components of the diet and least common in dairy farming areas.
Special clinical problems	Oxalate is an end product of several metabolic pathways—from ascorbic acid and glyoxylate found in the diet. People cannot metabolize oxalate, and renal excretion is the only route of elimination. Urinary oxalate excretion decreases with deterioration of renal function.
Dietary interventions	Avoid foods high in oxalate: tea, cocoa, beer, vegetables (beans, green leafy [collards, kale, spinach]), fruits (strawberries, purple grapes, rhubarb, cranberries, citrus peel), nuts (peanuts, cashews, almonds, pecans), and starches (grits, wheat germ). Increase fluid intake to maintain urinary output of 2 L or more daily.
Medications	
Phosphate	Decreases calcium oxalate supersaturation and stone formation.
Pyridoxine	Increases excretion of crystals responsible for oxalate formation.

Struvite Stones (Associated With Infection)

Incidence	About 15 to 20% of all stones are associated with infection.
Special clinical problems	Bacteria (usually *Proteus*) produce the enzyme *urease* that splits urea into two ammonia molecules; this raises the pH of the urine. The stones formed by this manner are *staghorn calculi* that grow to fill the renal pelvis and caliceal system. These stones are hard to eliminate because the hard stone forms around the bacteria, preventing the action of antibiotics.
Dietary intervention	Encourage acid ash diet: eggs, meat, poultry, fish, cereals, cranberries, prunes, plums, corn, lentils. Increase fluid intake to maintain urinary output of 2 L or more daily.
Medications	
Long-term antibiotics	To control infection.
Acetohydroxamine and hydroxyurea	Acid-urease inhibitors.

Uric Acid Stones

Incidence	Five to ten percent of all stones in the United States are composed of uric acid.
Special clinical problems	These stones tend to be the staghorn type and may be a consequence of (1) increased daily urinary uric acid excretion, (2) persistent concentration of urine, or (3) persistently acid urine. They are found in patients with gout, patients being treated for malignancy with chemotherapeutic agents or radiation, patients with chronic diarrhea, and patients with bowel disease.
Dietary intervention	Encourage alkaline ash diet: milk, fruits (except cranberries, plums, prunes), legumes, green vegetables; limit meats and fish, nuts (almonds, chestnuts, coconut). Avoid purine rich foods (liver, kidney, brains). Increase fluid intake to maintain urinary output of 2 L or more daily.
Medications	
Allopurinol	Used to prevent uric acid formation.
Sodium bicarbonate and other alkalis	To maintain urine pH at 6.5 or higher to decrease uric acid formation.

Cystine Stones	
Incidence	About 1 to 4% of all stones are composed of cystine.
Special clinical problems	Cystine is derived from dietary proteins. Acid urine aids in precipitation of crystals.
Dietary intervention	Dietary pattern is similar to that for control of uric acid stones. Increase fluid intake to maintain urinary output of 2 L or more daily.
Medications	
Sodium bicarbonate	Increases solubility of cystine.
Mercaptopropionylglycine	Decreases free cystine concentration in the urine.

(Sources: *Brenner and Rector,*[10] *Mahan and Arlin,*[44] *Tanagho and McAninch.*[79])

stone in the renal pelvis or upper ureter causes severe flank and abdominal pain accompanied by nausea, vomiting, diaphoresis, and pallor. A stone in the middle and lower segments of the ureter may cause radiating pain into the urethra in both sexes, into the labia of the female, or into the testicle or penis in the male. A stone in the terminal segment of the ureter within the bladder wall is associated with urinary frequency and dysuria. Intermittent pain usually indicates that the stone has moved. The pain may last minutes to days. Severe, sudden, and sharp pain is referred to as *renal colic,* whereas dull and aching pain may indicate early stages of hydronephrosis. Signs that infection is also present are chills, fever, and pain in the flank and back. Frequency of urination is common, but the urinary output may be decreased.

Diagnostic Studies

Gross or microscopic hematuria is usually present with any obstruction caused by a stone. If the stone is radiopaque, a survey film (KUB) of the abdomen will usually determine its general location. An excretory urogram is required to determine whether partial or complete ureteral obstruction is present.

Analysis of the composition of the stone is of utmost importance in planning treatment. All urine is collected and strained for analysis and measurement of how much sediment has passed through the urinary tract. A clean-voided midstream specimen is collected for routine urinalysis and culture for bacteria. Blood analyses for elevations of calcium, phosphate, and uric acid are also done initially.

Treatment

The primary goal of treatment is to preserve renal function. The patient with renal stones can be acutely ill. Elimination of stones may occur spontaneously; patients can pass ureteral stones 6 mm or less in diameter. Surgical intervention may be needed to remove large and intermediate-sized ureteral or pelvic stones (6 to 10 mm or more). Even if the stone is causing severe discomfort, the medical intervention may be a matter of waiting because most stones pass spontaneously.

Not all renal stones are alike and both treatment and recurrence are based on the type of stone formed. Certain stones form in acid urine, whereas others form in alkaline urine. Medications and special diets may be used to reduce the incidence of recurrent calculi. The achievement of the proper urinary pH may provide the highest degree of solubility for that particular substance. Table 48–18 provides information concerning dietary and pharmacologic therapies for various types of stones.

Mechanical and Surgical Interventions. The size, composition, and position of the stone in the kidney pelvis that does not pass will determine whether mechanical or surgical intervention is necessary. Laser therapy may also be used to remove ureteral stones.[43]

Mechanical intervention may be attempted. During a cystoscopy, a variety of special catheters with loops and baskets (Fig. 49–4) may be inserted through the cystoscope to manipulate or dislodge the stone. A ureteral catheter may be inserted past the stone. The catheter drains the urine trapped proximal to the stone and dilates the ureter, promoting spontaneous movement of the stone. The catheter may guide the stone downward as the catheter is removed.

In patients with large pelvic stones, a percutaneous tract may be made through the skin into a calix (*percutaneous nephrostomy*). The needle is guided by ultrasound (Fig. 48–11A). A nephroscope is used to pass instruments to pulverize and extract the calculi. After insertion of two catheters into the kidney pelvis, residual stones may be dissolved by percutaneous irrigation (*perfusion chemolysis;* Fig. 48–11B and C). Hemiacridin (Renacidin) may be used for struvite (infection stones). Other irrigants may be used for other types of stones.[79]

Extracorporeal Shock Wave Lithotripsy. Extracorporeal (means outside the body) shock wave lithotripsy (means crushing of stone) (ESWL, Fig. 48–12) is usually an outpatient procedure that permits removal of renal stones without direct surgical intervention. General or regional anesthesia or, in selected patients, local anesthesia is required; occasionally no anesthesia is needed. For this procedure the patient is placed on a table with a water cushion di-

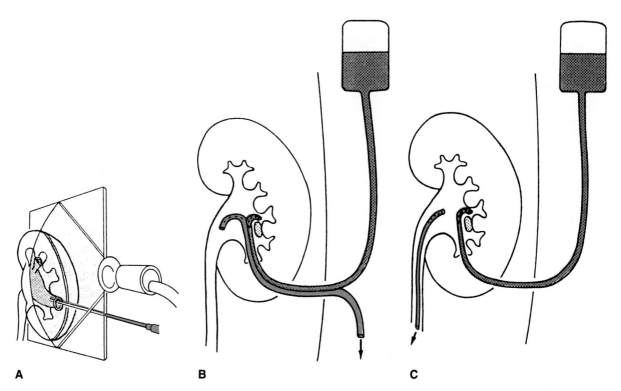

Figure 48–11. Percutaneous nephrostomy catheter insertion and perfusion chemolysis of renal stones. **A.** Guidance of needle (and subsequent catheter[s]) into lower calix by ultrasound. Irrigation fluid is perfused and drained (**B**) through two nephrostomy catheters or (**C**) through nephrostomy and ureteral catheters. (*From Tanagho and McAninch.*[79])

rectly under the affected kidney. The patient is "coupled" to the cushion by a gel between the cushion and the skin overlying the kidney. The kidney stone is located by fluoroscopy or ultrasound and displayed on the monitors above the patient and also at the desk. When the physician touches

the kidney stone on the desk screen, the computer automatically positions the rotating shock wave applicator and the table so that the stone is exactly in the shock wave focal point. To create the shock wave, stored energy measured in killivolts is discharged by electrode tips in the water cush-

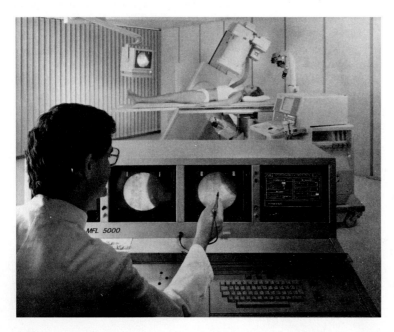

Figure 48–12. MFL 5000 Multifunctional Lithotripter. Patient is lying on table with affected kidney over water cushion; table can provide four-way movement. One of the monitors showing the image is seen in the upper left area. The rotating shock applicator that is shown at an angle behind the patient allows precise placement of shock waves to the stone. In the foreground, the physician is touching the stone on the computer, which will signal the computer to automatically align the shock wave applicator and the table so that the stone is exactly in the shock wave focal point (*Courtesy of Dornier Medical Systems, Inc., 1155 Roberts Boulevard, Kennesaw, Georgia 30144.*)

ion. The spark that is generated forms the shock waves that have a single brief pressure impulse on the stone measured in the nano- (one billion) second range. The waves can be transmitted through body tissue because of its high water content. Repeated shock waves, usually > 1,500, fragment the surface of the stone without damaging surrounding tissue. The numerous small particles pass spontaneously within a week in the urine.[79,86]

Calcium and magnesium–ammonium–phosphate stones have been successfully fragmented. Staghorn calculi may require a combined approach of percutaneous nephrolithomy to remove the bulk of the stone, followed by ESWL to pulverize any inaccessible fragments. Fewer than 10% of patients treated with ESWL have required subsequent nephroscopic or surgical treatment.[21,79]

If the preceding interventions fail, which is rare, *surgical intervention* is necessary to remove the stone. A *ureterolithotomy* is removal of a stone lodged in the ureter (discussed in Chap. 49). A *pyelolithotomy* is removal of a stone from the renal parenchyma. A complete end-to-end incision across the kidney may be necessary to remove an extensive staghorn calculus. There is very high recurrence of struvite stones unless all fragments are removed. An irrigation system with a stone-dissolving solution may be established. If kidney damage has been too severe, producing gross hematuria, pain, obstruction, and infection, a partial or total nephrectomy (removal of the kidney) will be necessary.

Complications and Prognosis

Complications include infection and hydronephrosis. The prognosis is excellent for a single stone occurrence but becomes less favorable if stones recur.

Nursing Management

When stones are causing obstruction, prescribed analgesics are administered to relieve pain, and antiemetics are given for nausea and vomiting. Warm baths and warm, moist heat to the flank may provide some relief. The patient should maintain a high fluid intake. Prescribed intravenous fluids are administered to maintain the urinary output if vomiting is severe. Fluid intake (from both oral and intravenous fluids) should be at least 3 L per day. Strict intake and output records should be maintained.

The urine should be observed for blood, and a decreased urinary output should be reported immediately. All urine should be strained and the degree of hematuria noted. Patients with renal stones may pass small, sandlike or gravel-like concretions with relatively little pain. The stone may not be in the form of a pebble. The patient should be kept as comfortable as possible using the measures listed earlier. Any signs of infection should be reported to the physician immediately, because infection will be treated rigorously with antibiotics. Patients should be encouraged to be as ambulatory as possible to facilitate passing of calculi.

Following ESWL the patient is instructed that hematuria will usually persist for approximately 1 week postprocedure. It is important to monitor I&O and to continue to strain all urine. Oral analgesics are prescribed for pain, and the patient should notify the physician if unrelenting pain, persistent nausea, vomiting, or fever is present.[74] All other aspects of care related to fluid intake and activity status are similar to those for the patient with urinary calculi.

When a *nephrostomy tube* is in place, the patient's vital signs are monitored frequently, because hemorrhage and dehydration from rapid diuresis of a relieved obstruction are possible complications. The urine is closely observed as to appearance and amount.[34] Transient hematuria is expected 24 to 48 hours after the insertion. The dressing is checked for signs of leakage around the tube, which may occur if the tube becomes obstructed. *It is extremely important for the tube to be properly anchored and to remain patent.* If the ureter should not be patent and the nephrostomy tube becomes kinked or occluded, damage to the kidney could occur from pressure. Kinking can be prevented by arranging 4 × 4-in. compresses around the site where the tube is inserted, and then taping the dressing securely.

Postoperative hemorrhage is a common complication following procedures to remove stones because the kidney is such a vascular organ. Thus, the patient should be assessed frequently for signs of shock. The hemoglobin and hematocrit should be monitored closely and the physician notified immediately if there are any significant decreases.

The care of a patient having a *nephrectomy* is similar to that for any surgical patient. Prevention of atelectasis and pneumonia is a challenge. Deep breathing and coughing are very difficult for the patient because the incision is so close to the diaphragm. Effective lung expansion needs to be promoted. Renal output is carefully monitored. The patient should be assured that adequate functioning can be maintained with one kidney. Paralytic ileus may also occur postoperatively. Bowel sounds are auscultated routinely and the abdomen is assessed. If no bowel sounds are heard or if the abdomen becomes distended, oral intake is withheld and the findings are reported to the physician.

The dressing and wound drains are monitored for serosanguineous drainage. Internal hemorrhage may also occur; the patient should be assessed for tachycardia, hypotension, dyspnea, restlessness, changes in mental status, cold clammy skin, and cyanosis. The appearance of any excessive drainage on the dressing that is frankly red should be immediately reported. The upper abdomen and flank area should be assessed for distention caused by pooling of the blood. The patient should be prepared for immediate surgical intervention and blood replacement should this complication occur.

 ## Discharge Planning and Community Care

Once the renal stone has passed or been removed and the patient is feeling better, he or she needs to learn about the diet, medications, and fluid intake. Fluid intake should be 3 to 4 L daily. The patient needs to be aware that some changes in lifestyle may be needed to allow time for fluid intake and urination. Although it is a fact that stone recur-

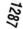

ⁿ, the hopeful aspect of this disorder should ⌐ by enumerating the measures that can be .tempt to prevent further calculi. The patient shou.ᵣ ᵢcouraged to express feelings and concerns. Early mobilization is encouraged to prevent urinary stasis and hypercalciuria.

A family member of a patient who has a nephrostomy tube will need to be taught how to change the dressing using aseptic technique; the importance of anchoring and maintaining patency of the catheter is stressed. It should be emphasized that follow-up care will be necessary and the need for this care is stressed in spite of the fact that the patient feels better. The principles under Nursing Management: Prevention and Reduction of Risk Factors may be reviewed when appropriate.

Evaluation/Desired Outcomes. The patient will:

1. Be able to verbalize the name, dose, action, frequency, and side effects of all medications
2. Understand and comply with fluid and dietary management of the particular form of stone disease
3. Be able to state signs and symptoms that should be reported promptly
4. Keep appointments for follow-up visits

■ RENAL CELL CARCINOMA

Benign tumors of the kidney are rare. This discussion is therefore limited to renal cell carcinoma.

Renal cell carcinoma (also called *renal adenocarcinoma* or *hypernephroma*) originates from the epithelial cells of the proximal convoluted tubules.

Incidence and Epidemiology

The incidence of renal cell carcinoma in the United States is 7.5/100,000 population per year. It accounts for about 2.3 and 1.6% of male and female deaths, respectively, from cancer per year. These parenchymal tumors constitute about 85% of all primary malignant renal tumors. The greatest number of cases occur in patients in their sixties, with twice the incidence in men as in women. A moderate correlation has been established with smoking.[10]

Clinical Findings

Very few symptoms are secondary to renal cell carcinoma. Many are nonurologic, such as weakness, fatigue, weight loss, and anemia. The classic triad of symptoms consists of gross intermittent hematuria; dull flank pain; and a palpable flank mass. Unfortunately, this triad represents far advanced disease and is seen in only 5 to 10% of patients at presentation.[10] Fever caused by release of pyrogens from the tumor, hepatosplenomegaly, hypertension possibly related to renin release, amyloidosis, and thrombophlebitis are also found. Vena caval obstruction by the tumor causes edema of genitalia and legs, dilated surface abdominal vessels, and ascites.

Diagnostic Studies

Because of the wide variety of presenting symptoms, the diagnosis of renal cell carcinoma may be suggested by radiologic testing. A survey film of the abdomen may show kidney enlargement or calcification. Ultrasound is helpful in determining whether a mass is solid or fluid-filled. CT and MRI may also be used. Renal arteriography provides direct visualization of the renal vasculature with a very high degree of accuracy in differentiating renal cell carcinoma from a simple benign cyst.

Blood analysis may show anemia due to blood loss or hemolysis or, uncommonly, erythrocytosis (hemoglobin 18 g, hematocrit 55%), possibly due to erythropoietin production by the tumor. Abnormal liver function tests (prothrombin time, globulin, bilirubin, and alkaline phosphatase) without metastasis to the liver, hypercalcemia, and hypophosphatemia may be present. Urinalysis will commonly show albuminuria. A chest x-ray and bone scan should be done to detect metastases.

Treatment

Renal cell carcinoma is treated by surgical removal of the involved kidney after making certain that the opposite kidney is normal. The surgical approach depends on the patient's age and the nature of the renal disease. Because the routine flank approach does not require entering the peritoneal cavity, this exposure is the most widely used. A thoracolumbar incision can be made when large tumors are present or when exploration of the vena cava is required because of extension of the tumor from the renal vein. Appropriate surgical treatment is a *radical nephrectomy,* which includes ligation of the renal artery and vein, removal of renal fascia and the kidney, and regional lymph node dissection. When the tumor is located in the renal pelvis, a *nephroureterectomy* is usually done, in which the kidney, ureter, and a portion of the adjacent bladder are removed, because of the tendency of transitional cell cancer to seed down the ureter into the bladder. A *partial nephrectomy* may be done if the disease is bilateral or if the cancer is in the only functioning kidney. If the malignancy is extensive, both kidneys will be removed and the patient will be placed on long-term dialysis and possibly evaluated for kidney transplantation.

The surgical specimen is classified utilizing pathologic staging to better evaluate treatment and prognosis.[10,79]

Stage I	Tumor is confined to the kidney; renal capsule is intact.
Stage II	Tumor has broken through the renal capsule and involves the perirenal fat.
Stage III	Tumor extends into the renal vein, the vena cava (IIIA), or involves the lymphatics (IIIB), or both (IIIA and IIIB).
Stage IV	Adjacent organs are involved (IVA) or distant metastasis is present (IVB)

The role of radiation therapy in the treatment of renal cell carcinoma is controversial. Some authors have reported that preoperative and postoperative radiation therapy can improve survival rates more than surgical management alone.[10] Others state that postoperative irradiation may decrease the incidence of recurrence of a local tumor in patients with gross residual disease, but it has no effect whatsoever on distant metastases.[79] No chemotherapeutic drugs are consistently effective for renal carcinoma. Preoperative arterial embolization may occasionally be done with large tumors; it causes infarction of the kidney and collapses the vasculature of large vessels, thus decreasing operating time.

Complications and Prognosis

About 30% of new patients with renal cell carcinoma have radiographic evidence of metastases when first seen.[79] The major postoperative complications of nephrectomy are atelectasis and pneumonia. Paralytic ileus and hemorrhage may also develop. The prognosis worsens in advanced stages of the disease.

Nursing Management

Nursing management of the patient with renal cancer includes general aspects of care needed by any patient with neoplastic disease. The natural history of renal cell carcinoma is often unpredictable. Once the patient has evidence of multiple metastases, a rapid downhill course can usually be predicted.

Discharge Planning and Community Care

Prior to discharge, the patient should be taught the signs of urinary tract infection so these can be reported to the physician if they should occur.

When visiting the patient in the community, the nurse should inquire about the urinary elimination patterns and the characteristics of the urine. The patient should be encouraged to eat a well-balanced diet to prevent weight loss and fatigue. When appropriate, plans for terminal care should be discussed with the patient and family.

■ RENAL TRAUMA

The majority of renal injuries are minor bruises. Depending on the manner in which they occur, renal injuries are classified as either blunt or penetrating.

Injuries from *blunt trauma* usually result from direct injury to the back, flank, or abdomen and are compounded by multiple injuries to other organs. They are frequently seen following traffic accidents when the kidney is forcibly pushed against a transverse process or is punctured by a fractured 11th or 12th rib. These injuries also occur when a person falls on the abdomen, flank, or back. The type of laceration involved can vary from a simple bruising without rupture of the renal capsule to a complete shattering of the renal parenchyma.

Penetrating wounds of the kidney are usually caused by knives, bullets, or shrapnel. Such injuries usually involve simultaneous damage to the intestines, liver, spleen,

or other vital organs; surgical exploration is essential. When the patient is in shock from blood loss, the situation is critical and surgical exploration is an emergency. Figure 48–13 illustrates various types of traumatic injuries that can occur in a kidney.

Clinical Findings

Gross or microscopic hematuria is the cardinal sign; but if the trauma does not involve the urinary collecting system, absence of hematuria does not ensure that kidney injury has not occurred. A blood clot obstructing the ureter can also obstruct renal bleeding. With severe lacerations, serious hemorrhage may occur with all the signs of shock. In such instances, a mass in the flank is usually present and accompanied by pain.

Diagnostic Studies

An excretory urogram to evaluate the functioning of the unaffected kidney should be performed before surgery to aid in the decision about removing the affected kidney. If the traumatized kidney is removed and the remaining kidney is nonfunctional, the patient will be left anephric. If the patient has two functioning kidneys, unilateral nephrectomy can be performed if necessary without endangering the patient's life or requiring that the patient maintain life on dialysis.

Treatment

If the patient is in shock following renal trauma, vital signs should preferably be stabilized before an evaluation of renal function is made and surgery is attempted. Decreased renal blood flow secondary to shock may unnecessarily present an altered renal function. Immediate blood transfusions will be administered.

The goal of treatment is to preserve renal function to the greatest extent. The need for surgery will depend on the

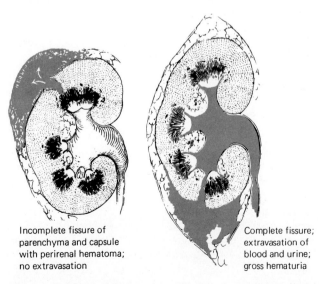

Incomplete fissure of parenchyma and capsule with perirenal hematoma; no extravasation

Complete fissure; extravasation of blood and urine; gross hematuria

Figure 48–13. Types and degrees of renal injuries. (*From Tanagho and McAninch.*[78])

level of traumatic injury. Contused kidneys often respond well to conservative treatment in which the patient is placed on bed rest (often at home) and the urine is observed for hematuria. Serial observations of the hematocrit and urine are made to monitor the progress of hemorrhage. The vital signs are checked frequently and an intravenous line is maintained to administer blood if necessary.

Penetrating injuries or continued moderate to severe hemorrhage frequently require surgical exploration to determine the extent of the trauma and to repair damage to the tissues. If the tissue trauma is too extensive, nephrectomy will be necessary.

Complications and Prognosis

In addition to the immediate problems of shock and loss of functioning renal tissue, kidney trauma can lead to a renal carbuncle, perinephric abscesses, and sepsis. Antibiotics are administered and the patient is monitored carefully. The prognosis depends on the extent of injury.

Nursing Management

The patient's vital signs and urinary output are carefully monitored. After the urine has totally cleared, the patient will be allowed to increase activity.

 Discharge Planning and Community Care

After discharge from the hospital, it is important for the patient to have follow-up radiologic testing to rule out any anatomic derangement of the kidney. The patient should be cautioned against driving a car or participating in any strenuous exercise or activity that would aggravate the traumatized kidney until the physician has approved such activities. During community visits, the patient is questioned about blood in the urine. The blood pressure needs to be carefully assessed to monitor for the development of secondary hypertension.

■ LEARNING OUTCOMES

After studying this chapter, the nurse will be able to:

1. Discuss major glomerular and tubular disorders.

2. Discuss the continuum of declining renal function. Differentiate among acute prerenal failure, acute postrenal failure, acute intrarenal failure, chronic renal failure, and end-stage renal disease with regard to the epidemiology, pathophysiology, clinical findings, diagnostic studies, treatments, complications, and nursing management.

3. Describe two types of dialysis and the related nursing management.

4. State the clinical indications for renal transplantation, types of potential kidney donors, tests for histocompatibility, complications of transplantation, and related nursing management.

5. Describe the pathophysiologic changes in the kidneys that may develop secondary to diabetic mellitus and hypertension. Explain the treatment and the nursing management.

6. Differentiate between acute and chronic pyelonephritis with regard to epidemiology, pathophysiology, clinical findings, diagnostic studies, treatments, complications, and nursing management.

7. Describe the major characteristics of adult polycystic kidney disease.

8. List common causes of urinary obstruction. Explain the pathophysiology of hydronephrosis. Discuss renal calculi including epidemiology, pathophysiology, clinical findings, diagnostic studies, treatments, complications, and nursing management.

9. Discuss the nursing management of a patient with renal carcinoma who requires a nephrectomy.

10. Differentiate between the various types of renal trauma and explain the nursing management.

REFERENCES

References for Chaps. 47 through 49 can be found on page 1311.

49

Disorders of the Ureters, Bladder, & Urethra

Christine Berding

CHAPTER CONTENTS

The function of the ureters, bladder, and urethra is to transport urine that has been manufactured by the kidneys and expel it from the body. Discussions in this chapter are related to problems that develop when there is infection, urinary retention, obstruction, or cancer in these structures, a neuromuscular disorder in the bladder and urethra, and trauma to the lower urinary tract. Excellent nursing care is of critical importance in monitoring the progress of these patients, observing for complications, and preserving functions of the urinary tract.

■ LOWER URINARY TRACT INFECTION

Urinary tract infection (UTI) includes primarily the clinical entities of pyelonephritis, reflecting inflammation of the kidneys in the upper tract (discussed in Chap. 48), and cystitis and urethritis, reflecting inflammation of the lower tract. Interstitial cystitis is a nonbacterial form of cystitis.

CYSTITIS AND URETHRITIS

Cystitis and *urethritis* refer to inflammation of the bladder wall and urethra, respectively.

Incidence and Epidemiology

UTIs are much more common in females than in males. At least 10 to 20% of the female population have a UTI sometime during their lives, and up to one third of elderly women have a UTI.[73] The incidence of UTI in males correlates with prostatic disorders, increasing from 4 to 10% in the elderly male.

1291

Nursing Management: Prevention or Reduction of Risk Factors

Nurses can provide the following information to female patients to assist in reducing infection.

1. Void whenever necessary so that stagnant urine does not remain in the bladder.
2. Be certain to wipe the perineum from front to back after a bowel movement. Bacteria in the feces can contaminate the urethra and increase the chance for infection.
3. Cotton underclothes are recommended. Underclothes increase perineal moisture which, when combined with the warm vulvar and perirectal areas, provide an excellent setting for contamination.
4. Drink two glasses of fluid before and after intercourse to encourage urination, which will assist in expelling microorganisms from the urethra. Void as soon as possible following intercourse.
5. Avoid bubble baths, perfumed soaps, and feminine hygiene sprays that may irritate the urethral meatus.

Pathophysiology

Organisms that cause UTIs in women usually colonize in the vaginal opening and periurethral area from a fecal reservoir.[73] The short female urethra provides easy access to the bladder, encouraging an ascending pathway for the infection. Indwelling urethral catheters result in UTIs in at least 25% of patients; they are the most prevalent nosocomial infection in the hospital setting. Bacteria enter the bladder by moving (1) upward within the lumen of the catheter from the collecting system or (2) up the mucous sheath and exudative material between the urethral mucosa and the catheter.

The urinary tract possesses some qualities that defend it against bacterial invasion. Organisms that constitute the normal urethral flora do not usually multiply well in urine. Extremes in urine osmolarity, a low pH, and high urea concentration inhibit growth of many bacteria. The flushing mechanism of the bladder is a very important defense mechanism. Urine flow dilutes the bacteria and voiding flushes them from the body. Any interference with normal voiding, such as obstruction or incomplete bladder emptying, can lead to bacterial retention and multiplication. Urine, bladder mucosa, and prostatic secretions have direct antibacterial properties.

Clinical Findings

The most common clinical findings in cystitis are frequent, painful urination in small amounts, suprapubic heaviness, and pain resulting from inflammation and irritation of the urethral and bladder mucosa; however, some individuals with bacteriuria may be asymptomatic. Urine may be blood-tinged or grossly bloody as a result of damage to superficial blood vessels in the bladder mucosa. The lining of the urethra may be red and irritated, and the lips of the meatus may be swollen. Fever tends to be absent. Within 1 or 2 days, upper urinary tract symptoms may appear as the infection ascends to the ureters and kidneys.[73]

Diagnostic Studies

Urine from healthy individuals usually contains fewer than 10,000 (10^4) organisms per milliliter of urine. *Significant bacteriuria* is defined as 10^5 or more organisms per milliliter of urine.[73] The diagnosis of UTI depends on persistent clinical symptoms being present and isolation of bacteria from the urine, usually with a urine culture. *Pyuria* (an increased number of white blood cells in the urine) and microscopic or gross hematuria may be present. Bacteriuria in a urine specimen obtained from a suprapubic tap (a sample of urine collected from the bladder with a sterile needle and syringe), a urethral catheter, or a clean-catch midstream specimen usually indicates that an infection is present.

Treatment

The goals of treatment are to rid the urinary tract of the invading organisms and to prevent recurrence of infection. Antibiotics are prescribed; effective therapy will result in a significant decrease in bacterial organisms within 48 hours of the onset of treatment. Topical antibiotics applied to the external urinary meatus may be included in the treatment of urethritis. Sitz baths may also be helpful. Any factors predisposing to infection, such as obstruction or calculi, are identified and corrected, if possible.

Forcing fluids has been advocated to flush bacteria from the bladder; however, it may hinder therapy by lowering urinary concentrations of antimicrobial agents.[73] Therefore, increased fluid intake may or may not be recommended.

An interesting *research study* has shown evidence that cranberry juice decreases the risk of recurrent bacterial infections in elderly women. Researchers found that women who drank 300 mL (10 oz) of cranberry juice a day for 6 months were 58% less likely to have bacteriuria and pyuria than those who drank a placebo.[5]

Complications and Prognosis

Cystitis may lead to pyelonephritis, as the infection ascends into the ureters and renal pelvis. This is an infrequent but serious complication. The prognosis depends on the severity of the infection and the general health of the individual.

Nursing Management

These patients are usually treated as outpatients. It is rarely necessary to hospitalize them, although cystitis and urethritis often develop in patients who have an indwelling Foley catheter.

 Discharge Planning and Community Care

The patient is instructed to take the medication exactly as prescribed, especially to take all of it. Fluid intake of at least 3 L daily may or may not be prescribed. Once the medication has been completed, the patient should be encouraged to drink at least eight glasses of fluid a day. The patient should be instructed to avoid sexual intercourse until the symptoms subside because of irritation of the urethra. Information about preventing reinfection, such as the preventive instructions supplied in this section, needs to be given. If recurrent infections are being experienced, the patient is asked if the infections are affecting sexual relations, which can be a common problem. The patient should be provided an opportunity to discuss this aspect of the experience and given support by listening and teaching the above information.

Careful follow-up is essential to determine the effectiveness of therapy. Many studies indicate that approximately 80% of adult females with bacteriuria have recurrent infection within 1 year, most within the first 3 months. The patient needs to know when to bring specimens and how to collect them.

INTERSTITIAL CYSTITIS

Also known as *Hunner's ulcer* or *submucous fibrosis,* interstitial cystitis (IC) is primarily a chronic bladder disorder that affects middle-aged women. It is a nonbacterial form of cystitis that results in decreased bladder capacity caused by inflammation and fibrosis of the bladder wall. Mucosal splits and small hemorrhagic lesions may also be present.[79]

The cause of IC is unknown. Many factors may be involved such as allergy, autoimmune disease, defects in or damage to the bladder wall, and obstruction to the vascular and lymphatic vessels of the bladder. Damage to the mucosal layer of the bladder allows harmful substances to penetrate the deeper tissues of the bladder wall causing inflammation and the symptoms of IC.

Clinical findings include complaints of severe frequency, urgency, nocturia, and pain in the bladder, urethra, and perineum, yet the urine is clear and free of infection. Hematuria may be noted by microscopic examination when the bladder is overdistended. Renal function tests and excretory urograms will be normal unless reflux has occurred. Physical examination usually reveals suprapubic tenderness. Cystoscopy confirms the diagnosis. When the bladder is filled with as little as 60 mL of urine, overdistention may occur. The mucosal lining of the bladder may split and bleed profusely.[48]

Treatment for IC is based on relief of symptoms; however, it may be prolonged and requires active involvement by the patient. Systemic drug therapy including the use of nonsteroidal antiinflammatory agents may help to control inflammation and relieve pain. Oral narcotics are occasionally used for analgesia. Anticholinergic drugs may help to relieve bladder spasms. In an attempt to enlarge the capacity of the bladder, hydrodistention with dimethyl sulfoxide (DMSO) is done at regular intervals, usually on a weekly basis. DMSO has analgesic, antiinflammatory, and muscle relaxant properties. *Complications* include gradual ureteral stenosis and hydronephrosis as a result of reflux; however, most patients respond to one or more therapies.

Nursing management includes establishing a supportive relationship with the patient. Discuss ways to modify activities of daily living to aid in maintaining an acceptable quality of life, such as installing a portable commode in a van to avoid frequent bathroom stops while traveling.

Teach the patient about the various treatments and encourage her to keep records of those used and their results. If hydrodistention is to be done in the home setting, teach her how to do it.[47]

■ URINARY RETENTION

Urinary retention refers to the retention of urine after it has been produced by the kidneys.

Epidemiology

Urinary retention may occur (1) following some surgeries, (2) from obstruction, (3) with some medications, (4) from anxiety, (5) from diseases with neurologic impact, and (6) following prolonged use of an indwelling catheter.

Frequent causes of retention in the hospital setting are certain types of *surgeries.* Intra-abdominal procedures, total hip replacement, spinal surgery, lower extremity surgery, hemorrhoidectomy, hernia repair, and vascular surgery are categories that most commonly necessitate postoperative catheterization.

The potential life-threatening cause of retention is *obstruction,* which most frequently occurs at or below the bladder outlet. Causes for obstruction may be attributed to intrinsic or extrinsic factors. Urethral strictures, prostatic hypertrophy, and bladder neck tumors are some common causes.

Medications that interfere with normal micturition and the function of the muscles in the bladder include anticholinergic–antispasmodic drugs such as atropine and belladonna alkaloids, belladonna and opium (B&O) suppositories, chlordiazepoxide (Librium), and papaverine; antihistamine preparations; beta-adrenergic blockers; and antihypertensives.

Many individuals develop particular rituals of voiding. Complete privacy, running water, normal position, and reading materials are common activities used to initiate the micturition reflex. When these factors are altered, *anxiety* may develop and produce muscle tension that may result in urinary retention.

Diseases with *neurologic impact,* such as diabetes mellitus, tabes dorsalis, and brain stem and spinal cord lesions, may cause neuromuscular disorders of the bladder, resulting in urinary retention.[80] The condition that results from these disorders is known as *neurogenic bladder* (discussed later). *Miscellaneous factors* include poor fluid intake and anorectal problems. Hemorrhoids or fecal impaction may cause retention by producing obstruction or inability of the perineal muscles to relax because of spasms.

Nursing Management: Prevention and Reduction of Risk Factors

Urinary retention may be prevented in some individuals postoperatively. Suggestions are listed in Table 49–1.

Pathophysiology

In acute urinary retention, the bladder does not suffer permanent pathophysiologic consequences once the urine is

TABLE 49–1

NURSING MANAGEMENT: PREVENTION OF URINARY RETENTION IN THE PATIENT POSTOPERATIVELY

Postoperative urinary retention may be prevented in some patients in the following ways.

1. Use the measures listed below to avoid the use of urinary catheters as much as possible, to prevent the dangers of urinary tract infection and tissue trauma.

2. Institute nursing measures to assist the postoperative patient in voiding. Allow the maximum amount of activity as prescribed by the physician and the patient's condition. Early physical activity increases the chances to void spontaneously.

3. If not contraindicated, have the patient in a normal position for voiding. Assist the *female* to use the commode at the bedside or in the bathroom. If she must use a bedpan, assist her to sit upright on the bedpan. Place protective pads under the bedpan to prevent soiling of the bed linens. Pad the bedpan with a towel to make it more comfortable. For the *male*, enlist the help of two assistants (preferably males) to support him to stand at the side of the bed to use the urinal. These may be the only measures necessary to initiate micturition.

4. Allow adequate time, because the urge to void may take several minutes. If possible, leave the patient alone. If the patient can sit up or stand to void, encourage increasing intra-abdominal pressure by leaning forward or pressing on the abdomen with a hand or arm to facilitate voiding, if this maneuver is not contraindicated by the type of surgery performed.

5. Encourage the use of relaxation techniques: close the eyes, take deep, slow breaths, and consciously relax the muscles, starting with the arms, legs, and then the trunk.

6. Run water in the lavatory, flush the toilet, put the patient's hands in warm water, pour warm water over the perineum, or stroke the inner thigh with light pressure. The running water may ease the patient's anxiety if the sound of voiding is embarrassing.

7. If none of these measures is successful, encourage the patient to rest and try again later. Provide reassurance by stating that most patients can void on their own. A positive attitude by the nurse often creates a positive attitude in the patient, thus facilitating relaxation and confidence.

8. Monitor the patient periodically for signs of urinary retention. Postoperatively, surgeons often prescribe to "catheterize if the patient has not voided in 8 to 12 hours." Take into account the amount of intravenous fluids administered since the last time the patient voided, amount of blood lost during surgery (amount is recorded on the operative note), and amount of distention detected when palpating the bladder.

drained. With chronic urinary retention, the detrusor muscle becomes hyperactive (causing frequency, urgency, and nocturia), which leads to muscle hypertrophy. The thickened bladder wall is more rigid and less easy to stretch normally, also leading to early activation.

In the postoperative patient with urinary retention, the inhibition of urination caused by anesthesia, drugs, or trauma in the region of the bladder depresses bladder sensitivity to distention. The impulses that produce the desire to void and the reflex emptying are not initiated. Other factors that contribute to urinary retention include the recumbent position, nervous tension, fear of pain, and spasms of the external sphincter.

Clinical Findings

Two cardinal signs of urinary retention are (1) absence of voided urine and (2) a distended bladder that can be palpated above the level of the symphysis pubis. Percussion of the suprapubic area may produce a dull sound indicative of a full bladder. A conscious patient complains of increasing discomfort and pain, which may be accompanied by increased blood pressure. A patient who is unable to communicate normally (endotracheal intubation) or is confused may be restless. If a neurogenic bladder (discussed later) is the cause of the retention, the patient may not sense the fullness of the bladder.

It will be necessary to differentiate urinary retention from oliguria or anuria, in which the kidneys are not producing normal volumes of urine. Patients having acute urinary retention have causes listed above. Patients who are unable to produce urine have conditions causing renal insufficiency or renal failure.

Treatment

Treatment is with catheterization or dilation of the urethra.

Catheterization. When all preventive nursing measures listed earlier are unsuccessful, a one-time catheterization using a straight catheter may be prescribed. If more than 500 to 1,000 mL of urine is drained from the bladder, the physician may request that a retention (Foley) catheter be left in place for continuous drainage. Usually, retention catheters are avoided as much as possible because of the dangers of UTI and tissue trauma. Even if intermittent catheterization has to be repeated several times, if strict aseptic technique is used, the chance of UTI or trauma to delicate urethral tissue is much less than with a retention catheter. Guidelines relating to catheterization are listed in Chap. 47.

Dilation of Urethra With Sounds, Filiforms, and Followers. Before a catheter is passed through either the female or male urethra, it may be necessary to stretch urethral folds and strictures, and also thread through difficult curvatures in the male. Instruments used are sounds, filiforms, and followers (Fig. 49–1). A *metal sound* is used to dilate the urethra; it is well lubricated prior to insertion. If this technique is not successful in the male, filiforms and followers are used. *Filiforms*

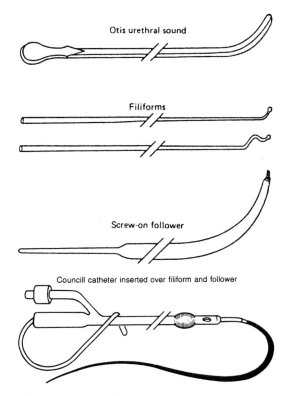

Otis urethral sound

Filiforms

Screw-on follower

Councill catheter inserted over filiform and follower

Figure 49–1. Devices to aid in catheter insertion. (*From Tanagho and McAninch.[79]*)

are soft tubes of very small caliber that can be used to probe for urethral openings. *Followers* are tubes of various sizes that have male connectors. These connectors are screwed into a filiform's female connector so that the follower can be passed into the bladder to dilate the urethra. Dilations are accomplished by removing only the follower, replacing it with a larger size, and passing it into the bladder. Once the urethra is dilated, a *Councill catheter* (similar to a Foley catheter but with an open tip) may be passed over the follower and filiform, and then the latter are removed.[79]

Suprapubic Catheters. If complete urethral obstruction is present and none of the above measures successfully drains urine from the bladder, renal damage may develop from reflux of urine into the kidneys. A *suprapubic cystostomy* (an opening into the bladder through a small incision in the abdominal wall) may be necessary so that a Foley, malecot (batwing), or pezzer (mushroom) catheter (Fig. 47–11) may be directly inserted into the bladder. Suprapubic catheters are used temporarily in association with bladder, prostate, and urethral surgeries and in acute episodes of urinary retention.

Complications

The bladder may distend to accommodate 1 L or more, possibly affecting bladder muscle tone. If this occurs, the bladder is unable to contract adequately to expel urine, resulting in urinary stasis.

Nursing Management. Mechanical dilation of the male urethra can be very painful. It is therefore important to request premedication for the patient if not already written. Postprocedure, the patient should be kept in a comfortable position; an ice bag to the urethra and analgesic medication as prescribed may help to relieve discomfort. If a catheter is present, it is not uncommon to detect hematuria initially following the procedure. The amount and presence of clots should be noted; if clots are present, the potential for obstruction of the catheter is a concern. Urine output is closely monitored. If there is no urine output or less than 30 mL/hour for 2 consecutive hours or the patient complains of bladder fullness, the catheter may need to be flushed, as prescribed.

The suprapubic catheter is taped to prevent dislodgement and is attached to a drainage system. If the catheter becomes dislodged, the catheter site should be covered with a sterile dressing and the physician notified immediately. Care of the patient with suprapubic drainage is similar to care of a patient with continuous urethral catheter drainage, as described in Table 47–9. The urinary output, along with signs of bladder distention, should be monitored. Suprapubic catheter tips may become mechanically obstructed by the bladder wall, clots, and sediment; methods of dislodgement are described in Table 47–9. If none of the measures is effective, the physician is consulted.

Hematuria is common for 2 to 3 hours after suprapubic catheter placement because of the incision into the bladder; then it gradually resolves. The degree of hematuria is noted at least hourly for the first 24 hours. The urine is examined for hematuria in the tubing before it becomes mixed in the drainage bag.

After surgery, a cholinergic medication such as urecholine may be prescribed to stimulate bladder contractions. It may be prescribed either before catheterization or after catheter removal. This drug is *contraindicated* when mechanical obstruction is present, because it increases intravesical pressure and could cause the bladder to rupture.

 Discharge Planning and Community Care

If muscle tone has been lost because of urinary retention, a bladder training program is indicated (discussed later). If an indwelling catheter is necessary to maintain urinary drainage, the patient needs to be taught the care discussed in Table 47–9 and signs of urinary tract infection that may occur following discharge from the hospital. When visiting with the patient at home, the nurse inquires about catheter care, palpates the patient's bladder, inspects the urinary meatus, and assesses the characteristics of the urine in the drainage bag. Problems related to the basic disorder causing the urinary retention are also discussed.

Evaluation/Desired Outcomes. The patient will:

1. Have the problem corrected that is causing the urinary retention

2. If an indwelling catheter is necessary, implement the correct procedures for maintaining continuous urinary drainage

■ URINARY OBSTRUCTION

Normally urine flows from the collecting ducts in the kidneys to the external urethral meatus. An obstruction may occur anywhere along this path, resulting in stasis or stagnation of the urine.

Classifications

Obstructions in adults are classified as to whether they are in the upper urinary tract (kidney or ureter) or the lower urinary tract (bladder and urethra). The obstructions may occur (1) within the urinary tract itself (such as ureteral and bladder calculi or neoplasms of the lower urinary tract) or (2) secondary to lesions outside the urinary system that compress or invade the urinary passages, such as prostatic hypertrophy. Other causes of renal obstruction are discussed in Chap. 48. Ureteral and bladder calculi are major causes of obstruction and are discussed in a separate section of this chapter. Urethral obstruction is primarily caused by prostatic hypertrophy.

Bladder Changes Caused by Chronic Obstruction

With chronic obstruction, such as with prostatic hypertrophy, the bladder may undergo changes in two stages: compensation and decompensation.

Compensation. During compensation, the bladder attempts to overcome increased pressure that has developed from the increased resistance to the passage of urine. The smooth muscle of the bladder (the detrusor) hypertrophies, sometimes to double thickness. The pressure during a detrusor contraction may increase from the normal 20 to 40 cm of water to 50 to 100 cm or more to overcome the increased outlet resistance.[16]

The normally smooth-muscled bladder wall may develop an abnormal, coarsely interwoven appearance known as *trabeculation* (Fig. 49–2). *Trigonal muscular hypertrophy* may occur, causing increased resistance to urine flow entering the bladder from the ureters. This produces back pressure on the kidneys which can result in bilateral *hydroureteronephrosis*. The increased pressure that is generated during micturition often leads to the formation of small pockets of mucosa that are pushed outward between the superficial muscle bundles called *cellules*. If the mucosa is forced through the musculature of the bladder wall, it may eventually develop into diverticula. These diverticula have no muscle wall and cannot expel the urine they contain, leading to stasis of urine, which predisposes to infection.[16]

Decompensation. Decompensation develops when the bladder tone becomes impaired or urethral resistance exceeds

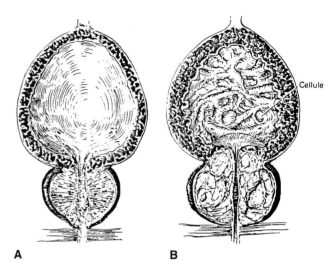

Figure 49–2. Changes in bladder developing from obstruction. **A.** Normal bladder and prostate. **B.** Obstructing prostate causing trabeculation, cellule formation, and hypertrophy of interureteric ridge. (*From Tanagho and McAninch.*[79])

detrusor strength. The contraction phase of the bladder becomes too short to expel the urine completely, resulting in residual urine. The symptoms of obstruction are pronounced: (1) urinary hesitancy, (2) need to strain to initiate urination, (3) small and weak stream, and (4) frequent urination. The amount of residual urine may increase to 1 to 3 L. Overflow or paradoxical incontinence occurs with the leaking of small amounts of urine from a distended bladder in the absence of effective contractions. The frequency of this leaking varies. Complete urinary retention may occur with no urine voided.

Ureteral Changes Caused by Chronic Obstruction in the Bladder

When trigonal hypertrophy occurs, damage to one or both ureters begins. The increased resistance to urine flow causes the ureters to dilate and hypertrophy near the bladder wall. The ureteral musculature thickens from increased peristaltic activity in an effort to push the urine downward. Bands of fibrous tissue may develop, resulting in bilateral dilation of the ureters and secondary ureteral stenosis at the ureterovesicular junctions. The ureters may become elongated and tortuous. Eventually the ureteral wall becomes weakened and loses its ability to contract.

OBSTRUCTION CAUSED BY URETERAL CALCULI

Ureteral calculi usually develop secondary to renal calculi. Peristalsis and gravity facilitate their passage into and down the ureter. Complete obstruction is rare.

Ureteral calculi occur more often in men than in women. They are rarely found in the elderly.[83] The same principles related to prevention of renal calculi are applicable as discussed in Chap. 48.

Calculus formation is discussed in Chap. 48. Certain anatomic sites at which the ureters are narrowed lead to obstruction: (1) at or just below the ureteropelvic junction, (2) where the ureters cross the iliac vessels, and (3) where the ureters enter the exterior muscular coat of the bladder.[71]

Clinical Findings

The major finding with ureteral calculi is the sudden onset of costovertebral angle (CVA) (Fig. 47–8) or flank pain that radiates down the course of the ureter and becomes severe within minutes. The pain results from hyperperistalsis in the ureter (so the pain may be intermittent) and distention of the smooth muscles of the renal calices, pelvis, and ureter. The patient may be tossing about and unable to find a comfortable position, or the symptoms may be variable with only a dull aching to CVA tenderness. The skin may be cold and clammy. Because of the similar neurologic innervation of the stomach and kidneys, it is not unusual for the patient to experience nausea, vomiting, and abdominal distention.[71]

Diagnostic Studies

A urinalysis usually reveals microscopic or gross hematuria, although hematuria may be absent if the calculus causes complete obstruction. Pyuria may be present with or without infection. The type of crystals in the urine may reveal the type of stone that is present.

About 90% of stones are radiopaque, and so they may be visible on a plain film of the abdomen (KUB) as a calcification in the area of the ureter. Ultrasonography and CT scans may be used to detect the location of the stone. If necessary, an excretory urogram or retrograde pyelogram may be used to demonstrate the exact location of the stone and resulting proximal dilation of the ureter (Fig. 49–3).

Treatment

The method of treatment depends on the size and location of the stone, presence or absence of a UTI, and the degree of symptoms. Indications for removal of stones include persistent pain, recurrent UTIs, urinary obstruction, and progressive renal damage.[71] Treatment may be expectant, by lithotripsy, manipulative, or surgical.

Outpatient Expectant Therapy. Outpatient expectant therapy may be chosen for stones less than 5 mm in diameter because they usually pass spontaneously. The patient is advised to remain well hydrated as evidenced by producing about 3 to 4 L urine daily and asked to strain all urine. Analgesics are prescribed to relieve the pain. If UTI and fever develop, the patient is admitted for manipulative or surgical treatment.

Lithotripsy. Large stones in the renal pelvis or proximal ureter may be removed with extracorporeal shock wave lithotripsy (ESWL), which disintegrates the stone with sound waves. Stones 5 to 8 mm in diameter usually pass

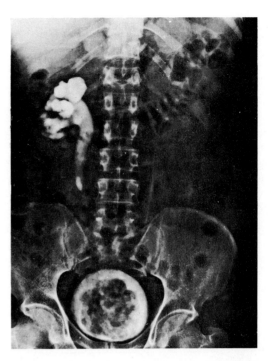

Figure 49–3. Excretory urogram shows a right ureteral stone causing hydronephrosis and a large irregular filling defect from unsuspected neoplasm in the bladder. (*From Way.*[86])

into the distal ureter and lodge in the ureterovesical junction. This location is ideal for transurethral manipulation.

Manipulative Therapy. With the use of cystoureteroscopy and fluoroscopy, stones may be moved and extracted. Balloon catheters may be used to dilate ureteral strictures and to aid in removal of stones. Guidewires and additional types of catheters may be used to guide instruments around the stone to extract it. One example is the wire basket (Fig. 49–4A,B). Small stones lodged in the upper and middle portions of the ureter may be removed using a ureteroscope with stone extractors.

After all the ureteral stones have been removed, the ureter may be intubated with a stent to prevent strictures while it heals. A ureteral stent (Fig. 49–4A) is a thin catheter that may be inserted into the ureter, either through a nephrostomy opening into the kidney pelvis to the ureter or retrograde through the urethra and bladder to the ureter. It may be curved on the end (into a "J" or a pigtail) to hold it in place. A guidewire is used for insertion and removal. The proximal end of the stent may extend through a nephrostomy, or the stent may be totally internal with the ends in the kidney pelvis and the bladder. The patient can be discharged from the hospital with the stent in place, and it can be removed 1 to 6 weeks after the procedure.

Ureteral stones may also be removed successfully by a percutaneous route. Under fluoroscopy or ultrasound, contrast medium is injected through a thin needle passed percu-

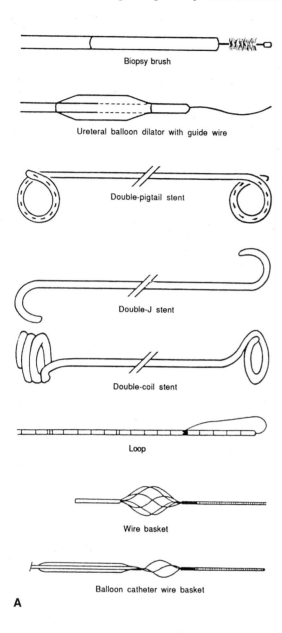

Biopsy brush

Ureteral balloon dilator with guide wire

Double-pigtail stent

Double-J stent

Double-coil stent

Loop

Wire basket

Balloon catheter wire basket

A

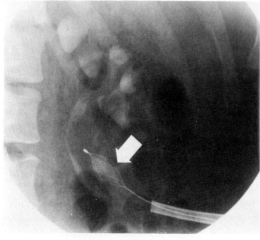

B

taneously into the renal pelvis to outline its boundaries. The medium may also be injected retrograde through a ureteral catheter to signify the location of the stone in the ureter; if obstruction is not complete, medium will flow into the renal pelvis. A small incision is made over the kidney area; instruments are used to enter the kidney pelvis or calices and then passed into the ureter to remove the stone.

Surgery. If the stones do not pass or cannot be disintegrated or extracted, surgical removal is indicated. With a *ureterolithotomy,* the ureter is opened to remove a calculus. With a *ureterostomy,* an opening in the ureter permits urinary drainage. These surgeries are indicated when the stone is obstructing the ureter and causing renal damage or is causing symptoms.

Complications

Complications from ESWL are discussed in Chap. 48. Complications resulting from stone manipulation include urinary tract infection, hematuria, ureteral perforation, breakage and entrapment of the stone basket, and complete avulsion (separation) of the ureter. The renal pelvis may be perforated, causing leakage of urine into the retroperitoneal space with a reduction in urinary output. These complications are rare.

The most common postoperative complication following a ureterolithotomy is urinary leakage. To avoid hydronephrosis from ureteral obstruction and edema, the ureter is frequently not sutured with a watertight seal. This leakage is temporary; however, leakage occurring more than 1 week postoperatively may be treated with a stent.

Ureteral stones that pass within a few days usually do not cause renal injury, but a stone that totally obstructs urine flow or is associated with infection may cause irreparable damage to the renal parenchyma or worsen a preexisting chronic renal infection.

Nursing Management

Prescribed analgesics are administered for flank discomfort associated with the presence of the stone and the procedures for removing it. Nursing management includes observing the patient for signs of shock and infection. The patient's vital signs and characteristics of the urine are monitored. Signs of infection include cloudy urine, increased back pain, chills, and fever. Oliguria or anuria may develop. Clots in the renal pelvis may occlude the flow of urine from the operative kidney. The patient is also observed for signs of pulmonary emboli caused by clot fragments traveling in the venous system to the lungs.

Drains that may be in place postoperatively include (1) a ureteral catheter, (2) a nephrostomy tube in the renal pelvis, or (3) a penrose drain or a suction drain such as a

Figure 49–4. **A.** Devices used for ureteral problems. **B.** Retrieval of stone fragment retained in inferior calix using a wire basket (arrow). (*From Tanagho and McAninch.*[78,79])

Jackson-Pratt drain placed in the tissues adjacent to the kidney and ureter. The ends may protrude through the incision or a nearby stab wound.

A nephrostomy tube may be left in place 5 to 7 days if no significant bleeding occurs. Gauze pads are arranged around the incisional drain to prevent the dressing from flattening the drain and obstructing the flow of urine from the wound. *It is extremely important that the tube remain patent because the renal pelvis holds only 5 to 8 mL of urine; obstruction can cause damage to the kidney tissue.* Montgomery straps may be used instead of tape to secure the dressing if frequent changes are required. Skin sealant should be applied to prevent irritation by urine. The urine should be blood-tinged to clear amber within 48 hours of surgery because the incision in the ureter is usually small.[45] The physician is notified immediately if the urine becomes bright red.

The incision may drain large amounts of urine for days or weeks after the surgery, so wound care includes frequent dressing changes. An ostomy bag may be placed around the wound to collect the drainage and to decrease the frequency of dressing changes. The site must remain dry (1) to prevent microorganisms on the skin from contaminating the incision and (2) to prevent the skin from becoming irritated.

The physician is notified if there is reduced urinary output, the patient complains of a feeling of pressure around the kidney, or the dressings become increasingly saturated with urine. These changes can occur with perforation of the kidney pelvis.

A foul-smelling drainage indicates a wound infection. The physician is notified and a specimen is obtained for culture per protocol to specifically identify the infecting organism and the appropriate antibiotics.

Discharge Planning and Community Care

The following aspects of care should be stressed. Additional information on discharge planning is presented in the section on renal calculi in Chap. 48.

- Encourage the patient to follow the prescribed medical regimen. Reinforce the information from the physician about the stone to which the patient is predisposed or actually passed. Include factors that contribute to its formation, such as dietary intake and urinary pH. State how the special diet and medications may help prevent further stone formation.
- If the patient goes home without passing the stone, advise to collect the urine in a glass jar. State that the stone will settle to the bottom of the container and must be saved for evaluation. This information will assist the health care team in providing appropriate treatment and preventive measures.
- Tell the patient that incisional discomfort and fatigue are to be expected for a few weeks postoperatively.
- Inform the patient to notify the physician if the following occur: chills, fever, flank pain, bloody urine, or changes in the incisional site that indicate infection (warmth and tenderness over and around the incision).
- If the wound is draining at the time of discharge, teach the patient or family member about wound care.

During community visits, the patient is evaluated for compliance with recommended therapies and for any recurrences of ureteral obstruction.

OBSTRUCTION CAUSED BY BLADDER CALCULI

Calculi in the bladder may result from (1) calculi formed in the kidney that have passed from the renal pelvis into the bladder or (2) calculi formed in the bladder. Bladder calculi may develop as a complication of urologic disorders that cause urinary stasis and chronic UTIs. A common cause is infection of residual urine with urea-splitting organisms, such as *Proteus.*[33] Breakdown products are crystals that can form stones.

Epidemiology and Pathophysiology

Nearly all bladder calculi occur in men between their third and fifth decades. Factors contributing to urinary retention resulting in urinary stasis and eventual stone formation include (1) bladder neck obstruction caused by prostatic enlargement, (2) bladder neck contracture, (3) urethral stricture, (4) bladder diverticula, (5) neurogenic disorder, (6) inflamed or ulcerated bladder, which may occur following bladder irradiation for cancer, and (7) introduction of a chronic indwelling catheter or any foreign matter into the bladder, which may act as a nidus (point of origin) for stone formation.[33] Stone formation is discussed in Chap. 48. The methods of prevention are consistent with the recommendations for prevention of renal calculi as discussed in Chap. 48.

Clinical Findings

A dull, aching, or sharp lower abdominal pain may be present with a history of hesitancy, frequency, dysuria, hematuria, dribbling, or a chronic UTI unresponsive to antibiotics.[71] With sudden occlusion of the bladder neck by a calculus, the male patient experiences a sudden interruption in the urinary stream with pain radiating down the penis. Voiding may be successful in a position, such as recumbency, that dislodges the stone from the bladder neck. This position may also temporarily relieve the pain.

Diagnostic Studies

The urinalysis reveals blood cells, albumin, and microorganisms. The diagnosis is confirmed with a cystoscopy, in which the stone can be visualized and the bladder evaluated for any pathologic changes. The type of calculi present is determined largely by the urinary pH and the concentration of stone-forming elements in the urine.

Treatment and Complications

Analgesics are prescribed for pain. Antibiotics are prescribed to treat existing infection and to prevent pyelonephritis. As a general rule, a stone that measures 5 mm or less in its greatest diameter has an excellent chance of spontaneous passage. It is often justifiable to wait for weeks or months for passage to occur except when (1) the stone is causing a high-grade obstruction that may result in permanent renal damage, (2) decreased renal function is evident, (3) infection is occurring behind the stone, or (4) the patient is experiencing pain that requires continual narcotic use.

Transurethral removal through a cystoscope may be used for a small (5 mm to 1 cm) bladder stone. If the stone is greater than 1 cm, a *lithotrite* (instrument to crush stones) is inserted transurethrally and the bladder is filled with saline. The stone is grasped in the jaws of the instrument and crushed; then the fragments are removed by irrigation. The stone may also be cracked using an *electrohydraulic* or *ultrasonic lithotrite* introduced transurethrally. An electric charge is delivered to the stone, fragmenting it.

Bladder calculi too large to be removed or crushed transurethrally may be removed through a *cystolithotomy* (a suprapubic incision into the bladder). The stone is removed and an incisional drain and urethral catheter are left in place for approximately 5 days. Urinary acidification to a pH below 6.2 may be helpful in minimizing precipitation of calcium crystals. Dietary modification can help to maintain acid urine (see Chap. 48).

The major *complications* are urinary retention, infection, and hemorrhage.

Nursing Management

Relief of pain may be obtained by (1) administering prescribed analgesics, (2) applying prescribed heat to the area, (3) providing comfort measures (Chap. 10), (4) using various relaxation techniques (Chap. 5), and (5) maintaining a nonstressful supportive environment. The incisional dressing may require frequent changes during the first 24 to 48 hours after surgery. Urine will be blood-tinged in the early postoperative period; an indwelling catheter is usually in place for 24 to 48 hours after surgery. The patient's urinary output should be monitored closely and the degree of hematuria noted. Any positive findings should be reported to the physician.

Discharge planning and *community care* are consistent with care of the patient with renal stones in Chap. 48.

Evaluation/Desired Outcomes: Obstruction by Calculi. The patient will:

1. Be relieved of the discomfort caused by the calculi
2. Have no complications from removal of the calculi
3. Comply with proposed preventive measures, such as dietary changes and increased fluid intake.

■ CANCER

CANCER OF THE URETER

Cancer of the ureter increases with advancing age and is rare in individuals less than 30 years old. It accounts for less than 1% of all genitourinary lesions. It affects men two to three times more often than women.[62] Epidemiologic factors are similar to those of other tumors in the urinary tract. Most tumors are transitional cell carcinomas.

Intermittent and sometimes profuse hematuria is the most common *clinical finding.* Pain from ureteral obstruction can occur over the kidney, in the flank, or as acute renal colic caused by the passage of blood clots in the ureter. Patients may also have symptoms similar to those of cystitis with fever, dysuria, frequency, bladder irritability, and back pain. Occasionally a mass may be palpated, which is a hydronephrotic kidney caused from ureteral obstruction.

Diagnostic studies include an excretory urogram, urine cytology, ultrasonography, and a CT scan. A cystoscopy is done when profuse bleeding occurs to determine its source; anemia is present with prolonged or severe bleeding.[12]

Treatment usually involves surgery. If only the lower third of the ureter is affected, a distal *ureterectomy* may be performed with ureteral implantation into the opposite ureter. If the malignancy is invasive or affects a site other than the distal ureter, a total *nephroureterectomy* (removal of the kidney, ureter, and attached segment of the bladder on the involved side) is performed. Chemotherapy is not effective for invasive cancer of the ureter. Radiation therapy is reserved for treatment of inoperable tumors. The *prognosis* varies with the grade and spread of the malignancy.

CANCER OF THE BLADDER
Incidence and Epidemiology

Bladder tumors are the most common of all the urinary tract neoplasms and the second most common genitourinary neoplasm (prostatic tumors occur more frequently). An estimated 52,900 new cases will be detected yearly in the United States. Bladder cancer accounts for at least 11,700 deaths annually. It is three times more common in men than in women and seems to affect Caucasians more frequently than African Americans.[3]

Cigarette smoking is the greatest risk factor for developing bladder cancer.[3] Studies show that the incidence varies with geographic location, with an increased incidence in areas of high industrial density. Coffee drinking and use of artificial sweeteners, such as cyclamate and saccharin, have been suspected as etiologic factors, but it is impossible to determine any overall enhanced risk.[22] Rubber and cable workers, textile weavers, dye workers, leather finishers, spray painters, hair dressers, and petroleum workers are reported to have a higher risk. Squamous cell carcinoma of the bladder is associated with chronic irritation and infection. Kidney stones and chronic indwelling Foley catheters have been considered to predispose the patient to developing this malignancy.[12]

Nursing Management: Prevention or Reduction of Risk Factors

Individuals who are at high risk because of their occupations should be informed by their employers, occupational health nurses, and through the public health department of the higher incidence of bladder cancer associated with their work. These individuals should consider eliminating other possible risk factors, such as smoking, artificial sweeteners, and coffee consumption, to reduce their exposure to possible carcinogens.

Pathophysiology

The pathophysiology of cancer is discussed in Chap. 11. Most bladder tumors are epithelial in origin.[12]

Clinical Findings

Hematuria is present in about three fourths of all patients with bladder cancer. The degree of hematuria does not correlate with the extent of the bladder cancer. Hematuria may be noted grossly in the urine or discovered only on evaluation for occult blood during a routine physical examination. Most patients have no other symptoms. Many times patients do not realize they need medical help until the malignancy becomes so advanced that an obstruction or fistula develops.

Diagnostic Studies

An excretory urogram performed initially detects rigid deformities of the bladder wall, ureteral obstruction that indicates deep invasion, other areas of upper tract lesions, and filling defects in the bladder (shown in Fig. 49–3). A cystoscopy determines the extent of the tumor on the bladder surface, and a biopsy is essential in staging the tumor. Accurate staging is the goal of all diagnostic tests.

Treatment and Staging

Treatment is based on the staging. The TNM classification by Marshall is summarized:[80]

- *Stage O.* Tumor is limited to the transitional epithelial mucosa and in situ carcinoma.
- *Stage A.* Tumor has invaded the submucosa but not the muscle of the bladder wall.
- *Stage B.* Tumor has penetrated less than halfway through the muscle wall or more than halfway but is still confined to the muscles.
- *Stage C.* Tumor has penetrated beyond the muscle layer into the perivesicular fat. It has not yet metastasized.
- *Stage D.* Tumor has extended beyond the bladder and perivesicular fat, but is still confined to the pelvis (D1) or has metastasized to distant organs or lymph nodes (D2).

Surgery. Superficial lesions (stage O or A) without muscle invasion are most successfully treated by excision of the tumor through the urethra (*transurethral resection*) with or without *fulguration* (destruction of living tissue by electric sparks generated by a high-frequency current). The patient may begin a course of chemotherapy with thiotepa instilled into the bladder. Follow-up with a cystoscopy every 3 to 6 months for several years is needed, because bladder tumors tend to recur. If the lesions have not responded in 3 to 6 months, other chemotherapies or intracavitary radiation therapy may be used. If the lesions continue, a radical cystectomy is performed.

A *partial or segmental cystectomy* may be necessary if the tumor (stage B or C) cannot be removed adequately with a transurethral resection. In the initial postoperative period, the bladder may only be able to hold 60 mL of urine; however, bladder tissue is very elastic and will soon stretch to accommodate the same amount of urine it could originally hold.[13] To prevent stress on the suture line, the bladder must be drained continuously through an indwelling suprapubic or urethral catheter. Meticulous catheter care must be maintained.

The treatment of choice for invasive bladder cancer is under debate. Studies suggest that the most effective treatment results from a combination of radiation therapy and cystectomy.[22]

A *total radical cystectomy* (removal of the bladder, urethra, and dissection of the pelvic lymph nodes) is performed if the bladder tumor is invasive. In the male the prostate and seminal vesicles are also removed, resulting in sexual impotence. Permanent urinary diversion is necessary for all patients. Radiation therapy and chemotherapy may also be used.

Urinary Diversions. Urinary diversions provide alternate routes for urine excretion from the body. They may be temporary or permanent, depending on the reason for the diversion. Malignancy of the bladder is the most common cause for surgery necessitating a urinary diversion. Other reasons include relief of ureteral or urethral obstruction, strictures, trauma, a neurogenic bladder, or severe damage to the kidneys and/or ureters from chronic infection.

The urinary diversions include an ileal conduit, continent bladder substitutes, cutaneous ureterostomy, and a vesicostomy (or a cystostomy) (Fig. 49–5). If no urinary diversion can be performed, *bilateral nephrostomy tubes* may be placed to provide direct drainage of urine from the renal pelvis. The nursing care for patients with nephrostomy tubes is discussed in the sections on calculi.

The most common permanent urinary diversion is an *ileal conduit,* in which the distal 6 in. of the ileum is ligated in two places; the portion of ileum retains its original blood supply. A standard bowel anastomosis is performed to reconnect the divided segments of the bowel. The proximal end of the conduit is closed and the distal end is brought through the abdominal wall as an external stoma. The ureters are anastomosed to the stoma and drain into it; a drainage appliance is required.

Continent bladder substitutes have been constructed. A *continent ileal conduit* developed by Kock[12,21] is similar to the ileal conduit except that it holds the urine until intermittent catheterization is performed. A nipple valve is created at the stoma by intussuscepting the terminal ileum backward into the ileal reservoir. As the conduit fills, pressure closes the nipple valve, preventing leakage. A *continent bladder substitute* may also be constructed from the ileocecal segment and placed in the abdomen. A reservoir may also be constructed from the ileocecal segment and attached to the urethra.

With a *cutaneous ureterostomy,* the ureter(s) is brought to the surface of the abdomen so that the urine

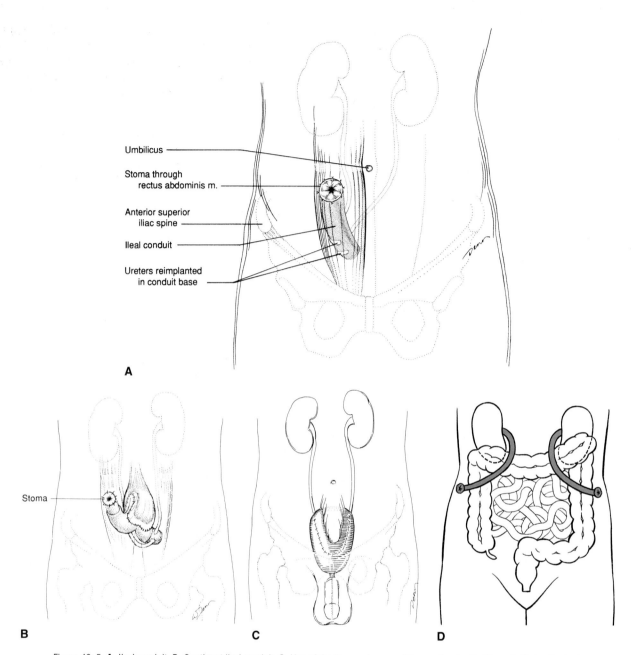

Umbilicus

Stoma through
rectus abdominis m.

Anterior superior
iliac spine

Ileal conduit

Ureters reimplanted
in conduit base

A

Stoma

B

C

D

Figure 49–5. **A.** Ileal conduit. **B.** Continent ileal conduit. **C.** Use of the ileocecal segment to construct a bladder substitute attached to the urethra. **D.** Bilateral cutaneous ureterostomy. (**A, B, C** from Tanagho and McAninch.[79] **D** from Norton and Miller.[54])

drains directly into a drainage appliance. The ureter-ostomy stoma is barely raised above skin level. The normal-caliber ureter has a poor blood supply distally, which may lead to the complications of stenosis or a compromised blood supply.

A *vesicostomy* is an opening made directly into the bladder. The bladder is sutured to the abdominal wall and a stoma is formed. Urine empties directly from the bladder through the stoma into a drainage appliance. A vesicostomy is needed if the lower portion of the bladder and the urethra are removed.

Complications and Prognosis

Complications of an ileal conduit include obstruction, leakage of the ureters, and vascular infarction of the conduit. If there is inadequate drainage, pressure can cause leakage of urine into the peritoneum. Edema at the uretero-ileal anastomosis can cause anuria. Late complications include stomal stenosis, pyelonephritis as a result of urinary reflux, renal calculi, and skin problems. Infarction of the conduit may not become evident for 5 to 7 days. Complications related to the ileal anastomosis include paralytic ileus, intestinal obstruction, peritonitis, and wound infection. The prognosis varies with the stage of the malignancy.

Nursing Management: Urinary Diversion

These patients have numerous needs that require comprehensive nursing management.

Psychologic Needs. Any sudden change in body image always arouses anxiety. Depression, withdrawal, and attention to body parts and functioning are expected during the grief period. Conclusions from a *research study* are that continuance of these behaviors beyond 1 year indicates a failure to adjust to an altered body image.[61]

The following are major ways to meet the patient's and family's psychologic needs:

- Develop an optimistic therapeutic relationship with the patient and the family. Realize that the patient is threatened by fears of separation from and rejection by the significant persons in the patient's life.
- Encourage the patient to look at the stoma and talk about the disfigurement or functional loss. Remind the patient that, despite the body alteration, he or she is the same person as before surgery.
- When possible, have the same nurse care for the patient during the hospitalization to promote continuity of care.
- Listen to the patient attentively. The patient may need to verbalize what has happened from the beginning of the symptoms. Tell the patient that it is normal to feel depressed, angry, and frightened.
- Be continuously supportive of the family and friends so that they can offer support to the patient. Discuss the postoperative altered body image and expected emotions and reactions of the patient with them. Tell them the importance of not showing disgust with the alterations.
- Provide information regarding a support group for the patient and family.

Preoperative Care. The patient is taught the importance of deep breathing, coughing, and leg exercises. Cardiopulmonary complications account for more than one third of postoperative morbidity and mortality with this type of surgery.[89] It is explained that (1) the lower bowel will be cleansed thoroughly as prescribed, (2) a low-residue or clear liquid diet will be prescribed, (3) antibiotics such as neomycin and erythromycin are usually prescribed for bowel disinfection to reduce the chance of infection from bowel flora, and (4) a nasogastric tube will be inserted on the morning of surgery.

The instructions provided by the surgeon are reinforced. The patient is taught (1) about normal anatomy, (2) how the urinary diversion will alter it, and (3) about the type of surgery that is planned related to the catheters, ostomy bags, stoma, and dressings. The patient is provided with a temporary pouch, adhesive products, and general equipment; their purposes are explained. Lengthy discussions about the specifics of care the patient will eventually need to manage are *avoided*. If possible, arrange for a rehabilitated person who has had the same surgery to visit the patient. If a pouch will be worn to collect the urine postoperatively, the surgeon and/or enterostomal therapy nurse determine the optimal location for the stoma. The stoma site must allow for thorough adherence of the pouch.

Postoperative Care. The patient usually spends the first few postoperative days in the intensive care unit following a urinary diversion procedure. Close monitoring is needed because a large amount of blood may be lost during an extended surgical procedure. Whole blood, packed red cells, or plasmanate may be prescribed to replace blood loss.

Care of the Patient With a Stoma With Continuous Urinary Drainage. Consult with the enterostomal therapy nurse to plan for and/or learn pouching techniques for the patient with a urostomy (Fig. 49–6). The pouching system is connected to closed drainage; the bag should be maintained below the level of the stoma at all times. Avoid tension on the tubing or the pouch. The pouch should be checked to be sure it is fitting properly. Stents extending from the stoma are noted; they preserve the patency of the ureter, which may become edematous and impede the flow of urine, resulting in increased intrarenal pressure and kidney damage.

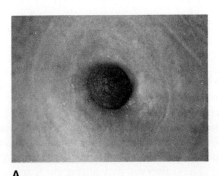
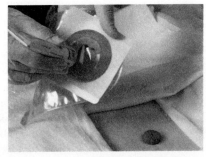
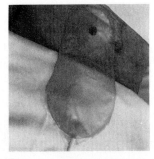

A **B** **C**

Figure 49–6. **A.** Well-healed urinary diversion stoma. **B.** Protective barrier applied to ring. **C.** Pouch attached to well-healed stoma. (*From Smith and Duell.*[68])

The urinary output is monitored hourly; output less than 30 mL hourly or any sudden change in output that is not proportional to the intravenous infusion rate should be reported to the surgeon immediately. Hematuria is expected in the early postoperative period, but the color of the urine should gradually clear to a normal yellow within 48 hours. Mucous threads in an ileal conduit are expected because mucus is a normal discharge from the ileal segment. Mucous threads should not be confused with pus, which will cause uniformly cloudy urine.

An edematous stoma is expected in the early postoperative period. The stoma should be examined every 2 hours for the first 24 hours and twice a shift for the next 2 to 3 days for any changes in size, shape, and color from the immediate postoperative baseline. The stoma should be moist and bright pink or red (similar to that of the mucous lining in the mouth). A dusky or cyanotic color should be reported to the surgeon *immediately*. This may indicate a decreased blood supply and the onset of necrosis, which is an emergency situation.

The skin adjacent to the stoma is checked for bleeding. If anything more than scanty bleeding is observed, the physician is notified. A small amount of blood may occasionally ooze from the stoma area, but continuous bleeding indicates that there are open blood vessels at the edge of the stoma.

In an ileal conduit, inadequate closure of the uretero-ileal anastomosis may result in leakage of urine into the peritoneal cavity. This complication causes a decrease in urinary volume in the appliance bag, boggy swelling around the stoma, prolonged abdominal distention with rebound tenderness, and signs of peritonitis (distended abdomen, abdominal rigidity, and decreased or absent bowel sounds). The physician should be notified if these findings occur. Edema at the uretero-ileal anastomosis may obstruct the urine flow, leading to anuria that usually resolves within 12 to 18 hours.

Additional Care. The nasogastric tube should be checked frequently and irrigated as prescribed by the surgeon. Inadequate drainage from the tube could result in pressure on the intestinal anastomosis and leakage of feces into the peritoneum. Intestinal functioning is assessed by listening for bowel sounds and carefully palpating the abdomen, noting whether or not it is soft, rigid, distended, or tender. Paralytic ileus immediately after surgery is a result of intestinal manipulation during the formation of the conduit. Peristalsis usually returns within 48 to 72 hours; the patient is asked if flatus is being passed. Any abnormal findings indicating urinary tract infection, such as fever, chills, or cloudy odorous urine, are reported to the physician.

 Discharge Planning and Community Care

It is of utmost importance to teach the patient and family every aspect of caring for the urinary diversion system. The patient's knowledge, ability, and readiness to learn are assessed. The aspects of care in Table 49–2 are important to assist the patient in self-care after discharge. The need for referral to a community health nurse or home health nurse is discussed with the surgeon. The patient who seems to be coping well in the hospital may do poorly at home.

While visiting with the patient in the community, the nurse assesses the stoma site and the urine and discusses problems the patient and family may be having. The need for an adequate fluid intake is reinforced. The patient is assessed for signs of metastasis (enlarged liver, anemia, or difficulty breathing). If these are detected, the nurse encourages the patient to contact the physician.

Evaluation/Desired Outcomes. The patient will:

1. Be able to change the appliance independently
2. Not be detectable as an ostomy patient in public
3. Maintain a satisfactory social and economic lifestyle
4. Return for follow-up visits
5. Maintain a urine output of 2 to 3 L daily

CANCER OF THE URETHRA IN FEMALES

Primary carcinoma of the urethra is rare in either sex but is more common in the female.[9] Cancer of the urethra in males is discussed under Cancer of the Penis in Chap. 65. Childbirth, coitus, or infection may contribute to the development of urethral cancer.

The *clinical findings* tend to be vague. Hematuria, urethral or vaginal bleeding, spotting, urinary frequency, itching, dysuria, difficulty voiding, and a palpable urethral mass may be present. Cytologic examination of urethral secretions and washings, urethrogram, cystourethroscopy, and biopsy are used to diagnose cancer of the urethra.

Treatment by partial urethrectomy or radiation therapy is usually successful in controlling localized lesions of the proximal one third of the urethra. Partial vulvectomy can be performed to obtain clear margins. Lymph nodes are examined to determine whether metastasis has occurred. Total urethrectomy requires urinary diversion. Carcinoma of the entire urethra may also be treated with postoperative radiation therapy and lymphadenectomy.

Nursing management includes providing psychologic support because the patient may feel a high degree of body mutilation from extensive surgery on her genitalia. Nursing management related to an indwelling catheter or urinary diversion is provided.

METASTASES TO THE BLADDER

Metastases to the bladder may occur from the prostate in the male; treatment is discussed in Chap. 65. Metastases may also develop from carcinoma in the intestine, producing an enterovesical fistula (Fig. 49–7). Clinical findings include *pneumaturia* (flatus in the urine) and *fecaluria* (feces in the urine). (These findings may also occur from a similar fistula caused by an infected intestinal diverticulum.) Treatment is surgery.

TABLE 49–2

TEACHING PLAN: THE PATIENT WITH A URINARY DIVERSION

1. Consult with the patient and the enterostomal therapy (ET) nurse to develop an education plan (teaching may be done primarily by the ET nurse).

2. If possible, arrange for a rehabilitated person who has had the same surgery to visit the patient postoperatively.

3. Encourage the patient to ask questions and to work toward independence at a comfortable rate. Provide written instructions.

4. Have the patient care for the urinary diversion as soon as possible postoperatively and continue the care until discharge.

5. Arrange all supplies and demonstrate use of the type of pouching system the patient will use after discharge.

6. Use the appropriate parts of Table 54–1 related to ostomy care. Teach the patient and/or caregiver how to perform the following:
   a. Use adhesive faceplate. The faceplate of the pouch is left in place 5 to 7 days unless there is evidence of leakage or skin breakdown.
   b. Remove the pouch. Carefully release the skin from the adhesive backing. Dispose of old pouch.
   c. Cleanse the skin. Use warm water only; soap leaves a residue that may interfere with tight seal of the faceplate.
   d. Apply the new faceplate and pouch.
   e. Empty the pouch when it is one third to one half full. Use a bedside drainage bag at night.
   f. Take care of the stoma.
   g. Control odors. Wash reusable pouches with soap and water, soak in dilute white vinegar solution 20 to 30 minutes, rinse with water.
   h. Detect problems. Report to the health care professional changes in color and odor of urine, significant increase or decrease in output.

7. Encourage fluid intake that will produce 2 to 3 L of urine daily to reduce the risk of urinary tract infection (UTI) and stone formation.

8. Maintain an acidic urine pH to prevent UTI, crystals on or around the stoma, and renal stones.

9. Review dietary factors related to urine odor. Asparagus, eggs, fish, and spicy foods can temporarily alter the odor of urine.

10. Teach how to prevent skin breakdown.
    a. Make a "wick" from gauze or a small soft washcloth or use a tampon to absorb urine that continually oozes from the stoma.
    b. Use warm water only to clean the stoma and the periostomal skin, pat the skin dry, and leave it exposed to air.
    c. Examine the periostomal skin for any signs of redness, breakdown, or signs of excess moisture. Only 1/16 to 1/18 inch of skin should be exposed between the stoma and the faceplate of the pouch. Note any yeast infection because of constant moisture. Apply nystatin powder, as prescribed, prior to applying the skin sealant and the faceplate.
    d. Apply skin sealant to the dry skin to prevent skin irritation from the adhesive backing of the pouch, tape, and/or moisture.
    e. Note signs of itching or irritation under the faceplate. Change the entire pouch, including the faceplate, immediately. Cleanse the skin as described above. Apply Karaya gum powder and skin sealant before applying the pouch. If skin irritation is severe, consult the ET nurse.
    f. Advise the patient to protrude the abdomen when applying the adhesive faceplate to prevent skin wrinkling and to promote a tight seal to prevent leakage. When the patient is in bed, attach the pouch "sideways" to support the pouch and facilitate drainage.
    g. Instruct the patient to use a continuous drainage bag at night.

11. Inform the patient of local sources of ostomy equipment and supplies. Encourage the patient to join the local chapter of the United Ostomy Association. The national address is listed in the Patient Education Resources. The focus of the group is to help members resume their normal lifestyle.

■ NEUROMUSCULAR DISORDERS OF THE BLADDER AND URETHRA

Neuromuscular disorders of the bladder and urethra refer to the inability of the bladder and urethra to normally expel urine, resulting in urinary retention, urinary incontinence, or both. Terms that are used interchangeably for these conditions include *neuromuscular dysfunction of the bladder and urethra, neurogenic bladder, neuropathic bladder disorder,* and *neurologic* (or *neuropathic*) *bladder dysfunction.* Because the disorder affects primarily the bladder, the term *neurogenic bladder* is used in this discussion.

Epidemiology

Many neurologic disorders, as well as other disorders, are associated with neuromuscular disorders of the lower urinary tract. Neurogenic bladder should be suspected in patients with diabetes, stroke, multiple sclerosis, trauma to the spinal cord, Parkinson's syndrome, and in those who are elderly.

Physiology of Micturition

For micturition to occur, there must be harmonious contraction and relaxation of the bladder and the urethral sphincters. The urethral sphincter consists of smooth muscle with autonomic innervation. Males also have an external sphincter, which consists of striated muscle with somatic innervation. When the detrusor muscle in the bladder contracts, it causes the urethral muscle to relax, which facilitates voiding. When the urethral sphincter contracts, the detrusor muscle relaxes, and micturition is terminated. All healthy individuals should be able to readily contract the urethral sphincter on command. If unable to do so, sphincter

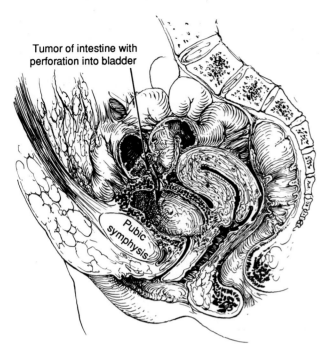

Figure 49–7. Enterovesical fistula caused by primary carcinoma of the sigmoid with perforation through the bladder wall. (*From Tanagho and McAninch.*[79])

dyssynergia, urinary incontinence, and urinary retention may develop.

Sphincter Dyssynergia. Sphincter dyssynergia refers to failure of the urethral sphincter to work in harmony with the detrusor muscle; there is inappropriate closure of the sphincter at a time when the sphincter is supposed to be open, causing urinary retention. The reverse may occur; the sphincter opens when it is supposed to be closed, causing urinary incontinence.

- If the urethral sphincter is *hyperactive,* it may contract when the bladder is contracting, producing outlet obstruction.
- If the urethral sphincter is *uninhibited,* it may produce sudden pelvic floor relaxation, resulting in sudden urgency or urinary incontinence.
- If the urethral sphincter is *inactive,* the pelvic floor will not relax at the time of attempted voiding and will obstruct the flow of urine.

Urinary Incontinence and Urinary Retention. A *hyperreflexive* (also called a *spastic* or *hypertonic*) bladder refers to a bladder with contractions that cannot be voluntarily suppressed. A *hyporeflexive* (also called a *flaccid* or *hypotonic*) bladder does not contract adequately and may result in urinary retention or incontinence. Incontinence is commonly seen in neurogenic bladder disorders. If a high residual urine volume is present, it may be caused by an inefficient urethral sphincter or a hyperreflexive bladder.

Classification of Neurogenic Bladder by Lapides

The most widely used and clinically relevant classification of this bladder disorder is the classification by Lapides (in 1970) into five types: (1) uninhibited neurogenic bladder, (2) reflex neurogenic bladder, (3) autonomous neurogenic bladder, (4) motor paralytic bladder, and (5) sensory paralytic bladder. This classification is based mainly on cystometrogram findings and does not use urethral disorders as a factor in classification.[88]

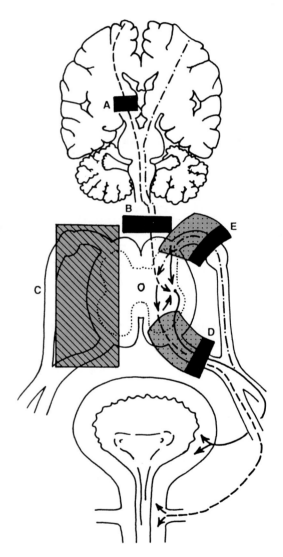

Figure 49–8. Types of bladder dysfunction related to level of lesion in nervous system. Sensory input is indicated by the —·— key. Lesions at point **A** or anywhere along the corticobulbar spinal tract produce *uninhibited neurogenic bladder.* Lesions that transect spinal cord above sacral level (**B**) produce *reflex neurogenic bladder. Autonomous neurogenic bladder* is produced by lesions that involve both limbs of spinal reflex arc (**C**), whereas *motor paralytic neurogenic bladder* occurs with lesions of motor cells or efferents (**D**). *Sensory paralytic neurogenic bladder* occurs when sensory efferents from bladder, dorsal horn cells, or sensory tracts to brain are impaired (**E**). (*From Mitchell et al.*[50])

Pathophysiology, Clinical Findings, and Treatment

The levels of lesions in the nervous system for each of these types are illustrated in Fig. 49–8. Table 49–3 summarizes the pathophysiology, clinical findings, bladder retraining methods, and adjuvant medications.

It is important to recognize that one form of neurogenic bladder may convert to another form during an exacerbation or recovery phase. For example, during an exacerbation of multiple sclerosis, an uninhibited neurogenic bladder may become a reflex neurogenic bladder.

The major goal of treatment is to preserve renal function. From the patient's point of view, the most annoying problem is urinary incontinence. When developing an un-

derstanding of the treatment of various forms of neurogenic bladder, the presenting clinical findings are considered. The presence of urinary incontinence, urinary retention, or both is noted; then the logical treatment modality is used. The treatment may include voiding programs, medications (listed in Table 49–3), and surgery.

Voiding Programs. Intermittent catheterization is preferred as a method for bladder retraining. Self catheterization is discussed in Chap. 47.

The *Credé-Valsalva method* involves the use of the patient's fist or palms of the hand to apply pressure over the bladder area while straining with the abdominal muscles. The

TABLE 49–3

SUMMARY OF NEUROGENIC BLADDER DYSFUNCTION AND MANAGEMENT TECHNIQUES

Pathophysiology	Symptoms	Physical Findings	Bladder Retraining Methods	Adjuvant Medications
Uninhibited neurogenic bladder[a] Defect in cortico-regulatory pathways	Urinary frequency, urgency, and uninhibited contractions	Sensation intact Bulbocavernous reflex normal	Timed voiding schedule	Anticholinergics to decrease uninhibited contractions
Reflex neurogenic bladder Lesion above S2–S4 segments	Involuntary reflex voiding	Sensation absent Bulbocavernous reflex hyperactive	Stimulation of reflex voiding through suprapubic tapping	Alpha-adrenergic blockers to decrease urethral resistance
Autonomous neurogenic bladder Lesion involves S2–S4 segments	Varies from constant urinary dribbling to overflow incontinence	Sensation absent Bulbocavernous reflex absent	Intermittent catheterization	Alpha-adrenergics to increase urethral resistance
Motor paralytic neurogenic bladder Lesion involves anterior horn cells and anterior roots of segments S2–S4	Ability to perceive bladder fullness but unable to initiate voiding May strain to void	Sensation intact Bulbocavernous reflex variable	Intermittent catheterization	Cholinergics useful in partial motor paralysis only, ineffective in complete motor lesions
Sensory paralytic neurogenic bladder Lesion involves dorsal horn cells or dorsal roots of S2–S4 segments	Inability to perceive bladder fullness but can initiate voiding May have overflow incontinence if chronically overdistended	Sensation intact Bulbocavernous reflex diminished or absent	Timed voiding schedule	Cholinergics to increase detrusor contractions

[a]*Types of neurogenic bladders as delineated by Lapides.*
(Sources: *Mitchell et al,*[50] *Tanagho and Schmidt,*[80] *Wein.*[88])

procedure is repeated every 30 to 60 seconds until no more urine is expelled. However, the use of the Credé-Valsalva method is *no longer advised* as a method to initiate voiding because of the potential damage to the upper urinary tract. Reflux of urine into the ureters and renal pelvis occurs because of the increased bladder pressure. In some types of neurogenic bladder and in the presence of vesicoureteral reflux, contraction of pelvic floor muscles increases the outlet obstruction and causes urine to ascend the ureters to the kidneys. This may result in hydroureter, hydronephrosis, ischemia of the renal parenchyma, impaired renal function, atrophy of renal parenchyma, and pyelonephritis.[84]

Patients suffering from incontinence caused by deficient external sphincter tone may be helped by a bladder training program using a timed voiding schedule (Table 49–4).

Male patients with extensive sphincter damage may be managed successfully with a Cunningham clamp, a padded clamp that fits over the penis. This may not be successful if there are excessive bladder contractions. Some patients may benefit from surgical implantation of an artificial inflatable sphincter (Fig. 49–9), which may be used in males and females.

Surgery. When a patient has a very small bladder capacity and has severe involuntary spasms of the extremities when voiding, surgery may be performed to convert the spastic bladder and extremities to a flaccid state. Surgeries include the subarachnoid block, anterior and posterior sacral rhizotomy, and selective sacral nerve section (division of the third sacral anterior [motor] nerve root). When the bladder then becomes flaccid, a bladder neck resection may be necessary. Approximately 1 to 3% of all patients with a neurogenic bladder require a urinary diversion because of upper urinary tract deterioration.

Bladder Pacemaker. Research continues in treating selected neurogenic bladder disorders with a bladder pacemaker. For neurostimulation of the bladder, levator ani muscle, and urethral and anal sphincters, single or multiple electrodes can be placed on selected sacral and pudendal nerves or their branches and then coupled to a subcutaneous receiver. The desired function of continence or evacuation can be selected; usually one or the other is needed in these patients.[80]

Complications

A patient with a neurogenic bladder usually has to live and cope with other medical problems. It is important to identify and prevent urologic complications so that the multifaceted problems do not become more complex. Major problems include urinary retention leading to urinary tract

TABLE 49–4

TEACHING PLAN: BLADDER TRAINING PROGRAM USING A TIMED VOIDING SCHEDULE

Teaching Principles	Rationale/Significance
1. Perform exercises to strengthen the perineal muscles (Kegel exercises).	1. Stronger perineal muscles can aid in controlling elimination of urine.
2. Maintain an adequate fluid intake (2 to 3 L unless contraindicated). Drink the fluids at regular intervals throughout the day and limit them in the evening.	2. An ample supply of urine must be present in the bladder to stimulate the micturition reflex.
3. Maintain a regular *timed voiding schedule:* on awakening, initially at 2-hour intervals, and at bedtime. Encourage the patient to increase voiding intervals to 3 to 4 hours.	3. A regular schedule can prevent overdistention of the bladder.
4. Do not try to void more often than every 1 to 2 hours.	4. Voiding too frequently leads to a reduced bladder capacity, thickening of the bladder wall, and decreased detrusor tone.
5. Initially keep a record of the times and amount of fluid intake and times of urinary output and whether continent or incontinent.	5. Maintaining records aids in determining whether changes need to be made in the amount of intake or times for voiding.
6. If overweight, reduce weight.	6. Weight loss may increase sphincter tone by decreasing pressure on the pelvic floor.
7. Avoid constipation.	7. Straining to have a bowel movement can decrease urinary sphincter tone.
8. Reduce impediments and delays when voiding.	8. Having a clear pathway to the bathroom and wearing clothing over the lower trunk that is easy to remove can prevent delay in getting ready to void.

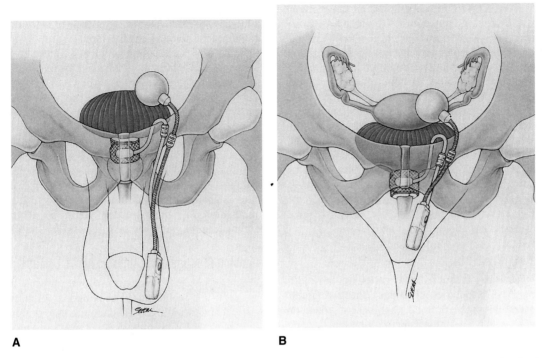

A **B**

Figure 49–9. Artificial inflatable urinary sphincter. **A.** Male. **B.** Female. (*Courtesy of American Medical Systems, Inc., 11001 Bren Road East, Minnetonka, MN 55343.*)

infection, urinary incontinence leading to skin breakdown, and a feeling of helplessness and embarrassment. Autonomic dysreflexia, which occurs in patients with spinal cord injuries, may develop; it is discussed in Chap. 39.

Nursing Management

All assessment skills are used in determining the patient's self-care functional abilities, disabilities, and desired and feasible health states. If the patient is unable to perform some of the procedures leading to bladder control, a family member or other individual must be willing to assist the patient. Most of the work to regain bladder control will be done outside the hospital.

 Discharge Planning and Community Care

Nurses generally determine the patient's limitations and needs once the patient is discharged from the hospital. A community health nurse is generally needed to continue guidance in implementing the plan of care. These arrangements need to be made while the patient is in the hospital.

■ TRAUMA TO THE LOWER URINARY TRACT

Trauma to the urinary tract is often overlooked in treating an accident victim for more obvious, often life-threatening injuries. When attempting to collect a urine specimen, the nurse may be the first person to discover that the urinary tract has been injured. Motor vehicle accidents are the major cause of urinary tract injuries.

Ureteral Injuries

Injuries to the small, mobile, elastic, well-protected ureters are rare. Gunshot wounds account for many ureteral wounds caused by external violence. Surgical injury may occur because of the close relationship of the ureter to the rectosigmoid and female reproductive tract. To prevent ureteral injury, many surgeons insert ureteral stents for better identification of the ureters.

When ureteral injury has been sustained as a result of surgery or trauma, *clinical findings* include flank discomfort, unexplained abdominal pain, fever, anuria, or kidney pain. Vomiting, a palpable abdominal mass, paralytic ileus, and sepsis may also develop. Leakage of urine through the vagina or surgical wound is an obvious sign that an injury to the urinary tract and adjacent tissue has occurred. If there is trauma that allows urine to leak into the peritoneal cavity, rebound tenderness will be present, signifying peritonitis. Hematuria is not always present, especially with transection, avulsion, and obstruction.

A plain film of the abdomen may reveal a large area of increased density caused by a large collection of extravasated urine. There is usually some degree of ureteral obstruction with hydroureter and hydronephrosis. An excretory urogram, ultrasound, or CT scan may demonstrate exsation of dye. A cystoscopy with ureteral catheterization and retrograde pyelography confirm the location of obstruction or leakage.

Treatment includes repair of the ureter with an end-to-end anastomosis if both ends of the ureter are healthy and if the ureteral ends can be rejoined without tension. Ureteral reimplantation into the bladder is frequently used to repair lower ureteral injuries. If reanastomosis or reimplantation is contraindicated, *transureteroureterostomy* (anastomosis of the injured ureter to the opposite ureter) is the treatment of choice when the ureter is not long enough to reanastomose, repair, or both. Stents are frequently used after repair to maintain a straight ureter with a constant caliber during early healing and to keep the ureter patent for urinary drainage.[79] *Complications* include stricture formation with resulting hydronephrosis.

Bladder Injuries

The urinary bladder may be injured by (1) blunt trauma to the abdomen when the bladder is distended (most common cause), (2) penetrating injuries caused by a gunshot wound or a fractured pelvis with bone segments perforating the bladder, or (3) attempted catheterization or urologic instrumentation.

A bladder injury may be classified as a contusion, extraperitoneal rupture, or intraperitoneal rupture. The *clinical findings* include hematuria if the patient can urinate. Gross hematuria occurs with bladder contusion. The patient may complain of suprapubic pain and being unable to void. The pain may increase over the first 18 hours.

With *extraperitoneal rupture,* which may be caused by a fracture of the pelvis, urinary extravasation is limited to the area around the bladder and does not extend into the peritoneal cavity or below the urogenital diaphragm. Lower abdominal tenderness and a "doughy" swelling may be palpated. If the urine is infected, cellulitis results. With *intraperitoneal rupture,* the trauma usually occurs in the lower abdomen. Bladder contents flow into the peritoneal cavity, resulting in lower abdominal pain, classic signs of peritoneal irritation, and shoulder pain (Kehr's sign). Chemical irritation to the bowel occurs if the urine is sterile; anuria may be the primary finding. Peritonitis results if infection is present.

A cystogram is the most dependable test to define bladder rupture. No specific treatment is necessary for bladder contusion. Extraperitoneal and intraperitoneal ruptures may be treated with an indwelling catheter, suprapubic cystostomy, repair of the bladder, and drainage of the perivesical space.

Urethral Injuries

Practically all urethral injuries occur in males. Contusion and partial or complete rupture may occur. Pelvic fractures frequently cause injury to the posterior urethra, whereas anterior injuries result from falling forcibly against or astride an object. Urethral bleeding, pain in the perineum and lower abdomen, abnormal position of the prostate on rectal examination, and inability to void are *clinical findings.* A tender mass may be palpated in the suprapubic area as a result of a distended bladder or extravasation of urine and/or blood. This extravasation may lead to cellulitis. The genitalia may be swollen or discolored.

A retrograde urethrogram will show the location and nature of the lesion. A urinalysis may reveal hematuria. The *treatment* of partial rupture of the urethra is placement of a suprapubic cystostomy catheter, urethral catheter, or both. A complete rupture may be repaired with end-to-end anastomosis.

A urethral stricture is a frequently occurring late *complication,* requiring reconstructive surgery. Penile fractures and injuries may result in damage to the erectile tissue, with subsequent partial or total impotence. Normal ejaculation is almost always regained after surgical correction of the urethral stricture, which frequently follows posterior urethral trauma. Penile implants are discussed in Chap. 65.

Nursing Management: Injuries to the Lower Urinary Tract

For all types of injuries to the lower urinary tract, nursing management includes (1) checking that all urinary tubes are patent and draining, (2) assessing the drainage, and (3) keeping careful records of intake and output. The patient should be monitored for signs of complications of infection, peritonitis, urinary extravasation, and abscess formation.

Traumatic injuries to the lower urinary tract frequently accompany other life-threatening injuries. During the acute stage, the patient may be overwhelmed with the medical and surgical care necessary to restore health. Once this initial stage is over, depression, anxiety, and withdrawal may occur. The patient needs to be encouraged to talk about his or her feelings. It may then be easier to look ahead and plan for convalescence.

 Discharge Planning and Community Care

On discharge, the patient is taught the signs of infection of the urinary tract with emphasis on the importance of reporting these to the health care professional. When monitoring the patient in the community, the patient needs to be questioned about any difficulty voiding.

■ LEARNING OUTCOMES

After studying this chapter, the nurse will be able to:

1. Discuss cystitis and urethritis as to the epidemiology, clinical findings, diagnostic studies, treatments, complications, and nursing management, including prevention and reduction of risk factors.

2. Describe the pathophysiology, clinical findings, treatment, and nursing management for patients with urinary retention.

3. Differentiate between the clinical findings in obstruction caused by ureteral calculi and obstruction caused by bladder calculi.

4. Describe the treatments used with expectant therapy, manipulative therapy, and surgical therapy for ureteral and bladder calculi. Discuss the related nursing management.

5. List epidemiologic factors related to bladder cancer.

6. Compare and contrast the nursing management for patients with an ileal conduit, continent ileal conduit, cutaneous ureterostomy, and a vesicostomy, which are formed in the treatment of bladder cancer.

7. Contrast the five types of neurogenic bladder, treatment, and nursing management.

8. Discuss the clinical findings, diagnostic studies, treatments, complications, and nursing management related to trauma to the ureters, bladder, and urethra.

PATIENT EDUCATION RESOURCES

Agency for Health Care Policy and Research (AHCPR)
The AHCPR publishes four resources on the topic of urinary incontinence:
Urinary Incontinence in Adults: Clinical Practice Guideline. AHCPR Pub. No. 92-0038.
Urinary Incontinence in Adults: Guideline Report. AHCPR Pub. No. 92-0039.
Urinary Incontinence in Adults: A Patient's Guide. AHCPR Pub. No. 92-0040.
Urinary Incontinence in Adults: Quick Reference Guide for Clinicians. AHCPR Pub. No. 92-0041.
These resources can be obtained at no cost by calling 800–358–9295.

American Association of Kidney Patients
211 East 43rd Street
New York, NY 10017

American Society for Artificial Internal Organs
P.O. Box 777
Boca Raton, FL 33432

Committee on Donor Enlistment
2022 Lee Road
Cleveland Heights, OH 44118

Help for Incontinent People (HIP)
PO Box 8310
Spartanburg, SC 29305
(800) BLADDER
HIP publishes a newsletter called *The HIP Report* and a *Resource Guide of Continence Aids and Services,* plus educational material. A nationwide support group was formed called *Continence Restored, Inc.* (785 Park Avenue, New York, NY 10021).

Innovations in Urology Nursing
Meniscus Health Care Communications
107 North 22nd Street
Suite 200
Philadelphia, PA 19103

Medic-Alert Organ Donor Program
1000 North Palm Street
Turlock, CA 95380

National Association of Patients on Hemodialysis and Transplantation
211 East 43rd Street #301
New York, NY 10017

National Institute of Arthritis, Diabetes, Digestive and Kidney Diseases, Division of Kidney, Urologic, and Hematologic Diseases
National Institutes of Health
Bethesda, MD 20205

National Kidney Foundation
2 Park Avenue
New York, NY 10016

The Simon Foundation for Continence
P.O. Box 815
Wilmette, IL 60091
1–800–23SIMON
The foundation publishes a newsletter called *The Informer.* Two support groups are a self-help program titled "I Will Manage" and an Incontinent Pen Pal Club titled Incontinent Pen Pals Yakking (IPPY).

Trio Transplant Recipients International Organization
1735 I Street, NW
Suite 917
Washington, DC 20006-2461

United Ostomy Association
1111 Wilshire Boulevard
Los Angeles, CA 90017

REFERENCES

1. Agmon Y, Brezis M: Acute renal failure: A multifactorial syndrome: pathogenesis and prevention strategies. *Moving Points in Nephrology, Contributions to Nephrology* **102:**23, 1993

2. Ahrens T, Prentice D: *Critical Care, Certification, Preparation & Review,* ed 3. Norwalk, CT, Appleton & Lange, 1993

3. American Cancer Society: *Cancer Facts & Figures—1996.* Atlanta, GA, American Cancer Society, 1996

4. Anderson S, Fedje L, Pulliam JP: Slowing the progress of renal failure. *Patient Care* **27**(20):102, 1993

5. Avorn J, Mondane M, Gurwitz JH, et al: Reduction of bacteria and pyuria after ingestion of cranberry juice. *JAMA* **271**(10):751, 1994

6. Bates B: *A Guide to Physical Examination and History Taking,* ed 6. Philadelphia, Lippincott, 1995

7. Berry L: Incontinence and urinary problems. In Carnevali DL, Patrick M (eds): *Nursing Management of the Elderly,* ed 3. Philadelphia, Lippincott, 1993

8. Borum PR: Nutrition support in pre-dialysis patients. In Wolfson M (ed): *Dialysis Reports.* Belle Meade, NJ, Cohner's Health Care Communications, 1994

9. Bracken RB: Management of carcinoma of the penis, urethera, and scrotum. In O'Donnell PD (ed): *Geriatric Urology.* Boston, Little, Brown, 1994

10. Brenner BM, Rector FC: *The Kidney,* Vols. 1 and 2. Philadelphia, Saunders, 1991

11. Bryan FA, Evans RW, Bergsten JW: *Home Dialysis Study: A Study of Factors Affecting Selection of Dialysis Treatment Locations: Final Report.* Research Triangle Park, NC, Research of Triangle Institute, 1978

12. Carroll PR: Urothelial carcinoma: Cancers of the bladder, ureter, and renal pelvis. In Tanagho EA, McAninch JW (eds): *Smith's General Urology,* ed 13. Norwalk, CT, Appleton & Lange, 1992

13. Chancellor MB, Blaivas J: Physiology of the lower urinary tract. In Kursh ED, McGuire EJ (eds): *Female Urology.* Philadelphia, Lippincott, 1994

14. Chandrasoma P, Taylor CR: *Concise Pathology.* Norwalk, CT, Appleton & Lange, 1995

15. Christensen J, Ostri P, Frimodt-Moller C, et al: Intravesical pressure changes during bladder drainage in patients with acute urinary retention. *Urol Int* **43:**181, 1987

16. Constantinou CE, Djurhuus JC, Yamaguchi O: Functional aspects of upper urinary tract transport. In Krane RJ, Siroky MB, Fitzpatrick JM (eds): *Clinical Urology.* Philadelphia, Lippincott, 1994

17. Corbett JV: *Laboratory Tests in Nursing Practice,* ed 3. Norwalk, CT, Appleton & Lange, 1992

18. Cummings JM, Houston K: The treatment of urinary incontinence. *Hosp Pract* **29**(2):97, 1994

19. Cunningham NH, Boteler S, Windham S: Renal transplantation. *Crit Care Nurs Clin North Am* **4**(10):79, 1992

20. Daugiradis J, Ing T: *Handbook of Dialysis.* Boston, Little, Brown, 1994

21. Donovan JF, Williams RD: Urology. In Way LW (ed): *Current Surgical Diagnoses and Treatment,* ed 10. Norwalk, CT, Appleton & Lange, 1994

22. Droller MJ: Transitional cell cancer: Upper tracts and bladder. In Walsh PC, Retik AB, Stamey TA, Vaughn ED Jr (eds): *Campbell's Urology,* ed 6. Philadelphia, Saunders, 1993

23. Evans RW, Blagg CT, Bruan FA: Implications for health care policy: A social and demographic profile of hemodialysis patients in the United States. *JAMA* **245**(5):487, 1981

24. Fantl JA, Wyman JF, McClish DK, et al: Efficacy of bladder training in older women with urinary incontinence. *JAMA* **256**(5):609, 1991

25. Fischbach F: *A Manual of Laboratory Diagnostic Tests,* ed 4. Philadelphia, Lippincott, 1992

26. Flynn JM, Hackel R: *Technological Foundations in Nursing.* Norwalk, CT, Appleton & Lange, 1990

27. Fretwell MD: Aging changes in structure and function. In Carnevali DL, Patrick M (eds): *Nursing Management of the Elderly,* ed 3. Philadelphia, Lippincott, 1993

28. Ganong WF: *Review of Medical Physiology,* ed 17. Norwalk, CT, Appleton & Lange, 1995

29. Garber AJ, Owen OE: Diabetes mellitus. In Stein J (ed): *Internal Medicine,* ed 4. St. Louis, Mosby, 1994

30. Greenspan FS, Baxter JD: *Basic and Clinical Endocrinology,* ed 4. Norwalk, CT, Appleton & Lange, 1994

31. Guyton AC: *Human Physiology and Mechanisms of Disease,* ed 5. Philadelphia, Saunders, 1992

32. Health Care Financing Administration: *Findings from the National Kidney Dialysis and Kidney Transplantation Study.* Baltimore, MD, US Department of Health and Human Services, 1987

33. Huether SE: Alterations of renal and urinary tract function. In McCance KL, Huether SE (eds): *Pathophysiology, The Biologic Basis for Disease in Adults and Children,* ed 2. St. Louis, Mosby, 1994

34. Jacobson HR, Stroker GE, Klahr S: *The Principles and Practice of Nephrology.* St. Louis, Mosby, 1995

35. Katz AH, Proctor DM: *Social-Psychological Characteristics of Patients Receiving Hemodialysis Treatments for Chronic Renal Failure: Report of a Questionnaire Survey of Dialysis Centers and Patients During 1967.* Kidney Disease Program, Division of Chronic Disease Programs, Regional Medical Program Service, Health Services and Mental Health Administration. Public Health Service, US Department of Health, Education, and Welfare, 1969

36. Kee JL: *Laboratory and Diagnostic Tests With Nursing Implications,* ed 4. Norwalk, CT, Appleton & Lange, 1995

37. Kellerman PS: Perioperative care of the renal patient. *Arch Intern Med* **154**(15):1674, 1994

38. King BA: Detecting renal failure. *RN* **57**(3):34, 1994

39. Kozier B, Erb G, Blais K, et al: *Fundamentals of Nursing: Concepts, Process, and Practice,* ed 5. Redwood, CA, Addison & Wesley, 1995

40. Lazaraus JM, Brenner BM: *Acute Renal Failure.* New York, Churchill Livingstone, 1993

41. Lehne RA, Moore L, Crosby L, et al: *Pharmacology for Nursing Care,* ed 2. Philadelphia, Saunders, 1994

42. Llach F: *Papper's Clinical Nephrology,* ed 3. Boston, Little, Brown, 1993

43. Mackety CJ: Lasers in urology. *Nurs Clin North Am* **25**(3):697, 1990

44. Mahan LK, Arlin M: *Krause's Food, Nutrition, and Diet Therapy,* ed 8. Philadelphia, Saunders, 1992

45. Marberger M: Percutaneous renal surgery: Its role in stone management. In Krane RJ, Siroky MB, Fitzpatrick JM (eds): *Clinical Urology.* Philadelphia, Lippincott, 1994

46. Martini F: *Fundamentals of Anatomy and Physiology.* Englewood Cliffs, NJ, Prentice-Hall, 1989

47. Melson G: Interstitial cystitis. *Ostomy/Wound Management* **39**(1):52, 1993

48. Miller JL: Diagnosis and treatment of interstitial cystitis. *Innovations in Urol Nurs* **5**(3):38, 1994

49. Mitch WE, Klahr S: *Nutrition and the Kidney.* Boston, Little, Brown, 1993

50. Mitchell PH, Hodges LC, Muwaswes H, et al: *AANN's Neuroscience Nursing.* Norwalk, CT, Appleton & Lange, 1988

51. Moffett DF, Moffett SB, Schauf CL: *Human Physiology Foundations & Frontiers.* St. Louis, Mosby, 1993

52. Morrison G: Kidney. In Tierney LM, McPhee SJ, Papadakis MA (eds): *Current Medical Diagnoses and Treatment,* ed 35. Norwalk, CT, Appleton & Lange, 1996

53. Newman DK, Lynch K, Smith DA, Cell P: Restoring urinary continence. *Am J Nurs* **91**(1):18, 1991

54. Norton BM, Miller AM: *Skills for Professional Nursing Practice.* Norwalk, CT, Appleton-Century-Crofts, 1986

55. O'Donnell PD: *Geriatric Urology.* Boston, Little, Brown, 1994

56. Palmer MH: Urinary incontinence. In Carrieri-Kohlman V, Lindsey AM, West CM (eds): *Pathophysiological Phenomena in Nursing,* ed 2. Philadelphia, Saunders, 1993

57. Peck P: Collagen injections put the squeeze on urinary incontinence caused by sphincteric deficiency. *Intern Med News and Cardiol News* **23**:3, 1993

58. Perryman JP, Stillerman PU: Kidney transplantation. In Smith SL (ed): *Tissue and Organ Transplantation.* St. Louis, Mosby, 1990

59. Price C: Issues related to the care of critically ill patients with end stage renal failure. *AACN Clin Issues* **3**(3):585, 1992

60. Price CA: Continuous renal replacement therapy: The treatment of choice of acute renal failure. *ANNA J* **18**:239, 1991

61. Reilly NJ: Advances in quality of life after cystectomy: Urinary diversions. *Innovations in Urol Nurs* **5**(2):17, 1994

62. Reilly NJ, Tomaselli N: Caring for a urinary diversion. *Innovations in Urol Nurs* **5**(2):23, 1994

63. Reischman F, Levy NB: Problems in adaptation to maintenance hemodialysis: A four year study of 25 patients. *Arch Int Med* **130**:859, 1972

64. Rose BD, Rennke HG: *Renal Pathophysiology—The Essentials.* St. Louis, Mosby, 1994

65. Schrier RW, Gottschalk CW: *Diseases of the Kidney,* Vols. 1, 2, and 3. Boston, Little, Brown, 1993

66. Sherwood L: *Human Physiology from Cells to Systems.* Minneapolis, West Publishing Company, 1993

66a. Slavis SA, Novick AC, Steinmuller DR, et al: Outcome of renal transplantation in patients with functioning graft for 20 years or more. *J Urol* **144**(1):20, 1990

67. Smith DR: *General Urology,* ed 11. Los Altos, CA, Lange, 1984

68. Smith SF, Duell D: *Clinical Nursing Skills,* ed 3. Norwalk, CT, Appleton & Lange, 1992

69. Snell RS, Smith MS: *Clinical Anatomy for Emergency Medicine.* St. Louis, Mosby, 1993

70. Sotolongo JP: Causes and treatment of neurogenic bladder dysfunction. In Krane RJ, Siroky MB, Fitzpatrick JM (eds): *Clinical Urology.* Philadelphia, Lippincott, 1994

71. Spirnak JP, Resnick MI: Urinary stones. In Tanagho EA, McAninch JW (eds): *Smith's General Urology,* ed 13. Los Altos, CA, Lange, 1992

72. Stark J: Dialysis options in the critically ill patient: Hemodialysis, peritoneal dialysis, and continuous renal replacement therapy. *Crit Care Nurs Q* **14**(4):40, 1992

73. Stein JH (ed): *Internal Medicine,* ed 4. St. Louis, Mosby, 1994

74. Stoller ML: Extracorporeal shock wave lithotripsy. In Tanagho EA, McAninch JW (eds): *Smith's General Urology,* ed 13. Norwalk, CT, Appleton & Lange, 1992

75. Strohschein B, Caruso D, Grene K: Continuous venovenous hemodialysis. *Am J Crit Care* **3**(2):92, 1994

76. Swan SK, Bennett WM: Nephrotoxic acute renal failure. In Lazarus JM, Brenner BM (eds): *Acute Renal Failure,* ed 3. New York, Churchill Livingstone, 1993

77. Talbot LA: Coping with urinary incontinence: A conceptualization of the process. *Ostomy/Wound Management* **40**(2):28, 1994

78. Tanagho EA, McAninch JW: *Smith's General Urology,* ed 12. Norwalk, CT, Appleton & Lange, 1988

79. Tanagho EA, McAninch JW: *Smith's General Urology,* ed 14. Norwalk, CT, Appleton & Lange, 1995

80. Tanagho EA, Schmidt RA: Neuropathic bladder disorders. In Tanagho EA, McAninch JW (eds): *Smith's General Urology,* ed 13. Norwalk, CT, Appleton & Lange, 1992

81. Tisher CC, Brenner BM: *Renal Pathology and Functional Correlations,* Vols. 1 and 2. Philadelphia, Lippincott, 1994

82. *United States Renal Data System Annual Report.* The National Institutes of Health, The National Institutes of Diabetes and Digestive and Kidney Diseases, Division of Kidney, Urologic, and Hematologic Diseases. Bethesda, MD, 1994

83. Walsh PC, Retir AB, Stamey TA, Vaughan ED (eds): *Campbell's Urology.* Philadelphia, Saunders, 1992

84. Walter MD: Retropubic repair of urethral incontinence. In Kursh ED, McGuire EJ (eds): *Female Urology.* Philadelphia, Lippincott, 1994

85. Wardle EN: Acute renal failure and multiorgan failure. *Nephron* **66**:380, 1994

86. Way LA: *Current Surgical Diagnosis & Treatment,* ed 10. Norwalk, CT, Appleton & Lange, 1994

87. Weber-Jones JE: Performing clean intermittent self-catheterization. *Nursing 91* **21**(8):56, 1991

88. Wein AJ: Neuropathic bladder dysfunction of the lower urinary tract. In Walsh PC, Retik AB, Stamey TA, et al (eds): *Campbell's Urology,* ed 6. Philadelphia, Saunders, 1992

89. Yeston NS, Grotz RL, Kantor WN: Preoperative and postoperative care. In Krane RJ, Siroky MB, Fitzpatrick JM (eds): *Clinical Urology.* Philadelphia, Lippincott, 1994